Healing
Back

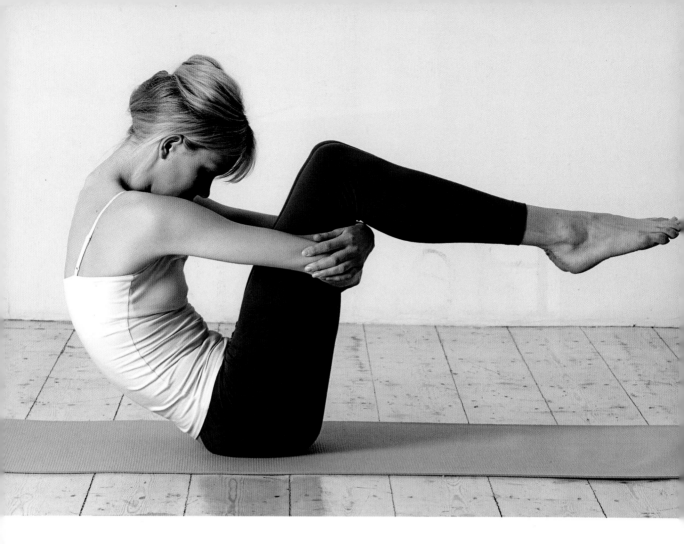

First published in the United Kingdom in 2008 by
Collins & Brown
10 Southcombe Street
London
W14 0RA

An imprint of Anova Books Company Ltd

ISBN 978-1-84340-432-3

A CIP catalogue for this book is available from
the British Library.

9 8 7 6 5 4 3 2 1

Reproduction by Rival Colour Ltd, UK
Printed by Craft Print Ltd, Singapore

This book can be ordered direct from the publisher.
Contact the marketing department, but try your
bookshop first.

www.anovabooks.com

Dedication
To Walter
with much love and gratitude

Notice to Readers
This book should not be used as a substitute for qualified
medical advice. While the advice and information in it
are believed to be accurate, neither the author nor the
publishers will be held responsible for any errors or
omissions that may be found in the text, or any actions
that may be taken by a reader relying on information
in the text, which are taken at the reader's own risk.

Healing Back

A practical approach to healing common back ailments

Stella Weller

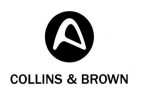

COLLINS & BROWN

Contents

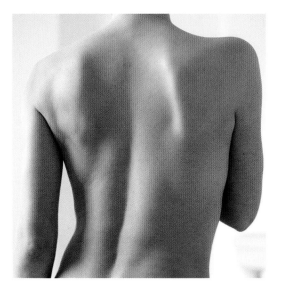 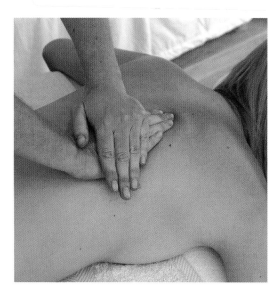

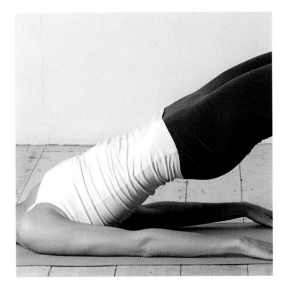 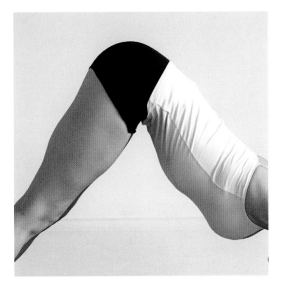

Chapter 5

Chapter 6

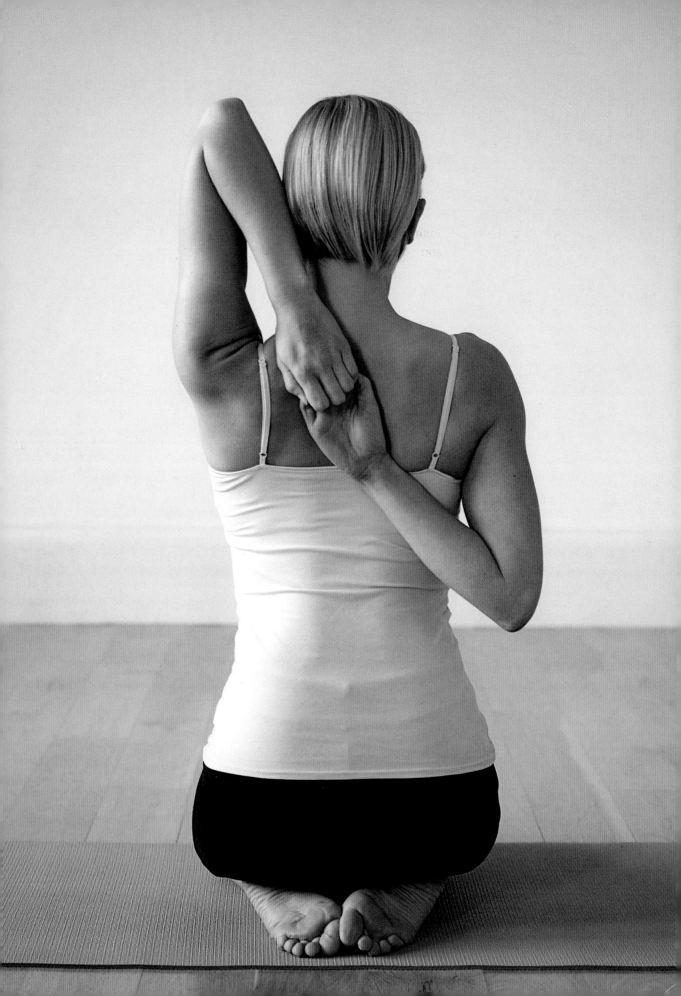

Introduction

The problem of back and neck pain continues to grow and has now reached epidemic proportions in the UK, America and many other countries. Statistics support the enormity of its impact on productivity and finances, but the costs in terms of human suffering are immeasurable. *Healing Back* explores what underlies back and neck pain and related symptoms, the various ways of coping with these causes and strategies to promote healing.

The first chapter, Background on the Spine, presents a brief and straightforward overview of the structure and functions of the spine and associated structures. Even a cursory reading will be well worth your while. It will help you to appreciate what can go wrong and why, and also the rationale for the measures suggested to help prevent certain problems from arising.

In What Can Go Wrong we look at the many departures from normal functioning that can occur in various spinal structures, and learn about some common tests and procedures used by health-care personnel to identify these disorders or to assist them in planning treatments.

Coping With Pain explores why pain occurs and the numerous ways of dealing with it, including methods you can try without professional assistance.

You will learn, or be reminded of, the significance of good posture in Posture Matters, and the impact on spinal health of persisting in bad habits when carrying out everyday activities. We also look at ways in which to correct poor habits and so minimise wear and tear on spinal components.

Exercises to help heal back ailments and prevent their occurrence are the focus of our next chapter, Healing Back Exercises. Two 'healing' sequences are offered, in addition to warm-up and cool-down sessions. Also included in this chapter is a reminder of why stretching is so important, and how you can add fun to your exercise programme through the use of a Swiss ball.

Finally, Ailments and Healing Options has information on more than eighteen common ailments that can arise from injury, disease or degeneration of the spine and related tissues: what they are, their symptoms and causes, preventive measures and treatments, both non-surgical and surgical.

Whether you're one of the few fortunate people who have never experienced a back problem, or one of the many who at some time have had to cope with backache or another spine-related ailment, *Healing Back* will be of interest to you. It may, in fact, be the only guide you'll need in your quest for a strong, healthy, problem-free back.

Spinal bones

The spine is composed of 33 bones called vertebrae (singular: vertebra). Of these, seven are cervical (neck), twelve are thoracic (chest or mid-back) and five are lumbar (in the loins or lower back). Five are fused into one bone called the sacrum (sacred bone) and the remaining four, known as the coccyx (resembling a cuckoo's bill), are fused to form a single bone. The upper 24 bones are movable, whereas those composing the sacrum and coccyx are not.

Spinal curves

When viewed from the side, the spine shows four normal curves. The cervical and lumbar curves bulge forwards and the thoracic and sacral curves cup inwards. These curves are important: they increase the strength of the spine, help us to maintain balance when we are in an upright position, absorb shock when we walk and help to protect the spine from fractures.

A typical vertebra

With some variations according to the part of the spine they occupy, vertebrae typically consist of a body, a vertebral (or neural) arch and several processes (projections).

The body, which is the weight-bearing part, forms the front of the vertebra. Its upper and lower surfaces (end plates) are roughened to accommodate the attachment of spinal (intervertebral) discs. The front and sides contain openings for blood vessels.

The vertebral arch is composed of two short, thick pedicles projecting backwards to unite with laminae (bony plates), which are flat.

The processes, seven in number, arise from the vertebral arch. They consist of one transverse process on each side and a single spinous process. These act as levers to which muscles are attached by tendons. The remaining four processes form joints, with vertebrae above and below.

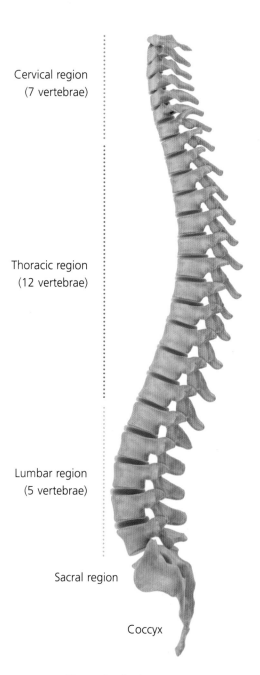

Cervical region
(7 vertebrae)

Thoracic region
(12 vertebrae)

Lumbar region
(5 vertebrae)

Sacral region

Coccyx

Normal spinal curves

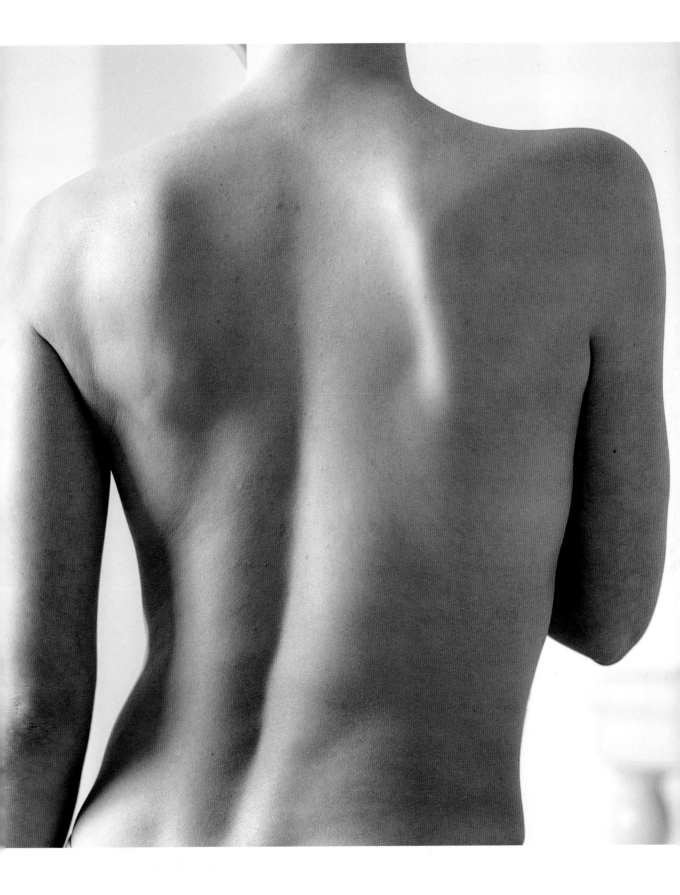

Spinal nerves

Contained within the bony canal that runs the entire length of the spine are the spinal cord and nerves. Between the bones that form the spine are openings (foramina) for the passage of nerves, which connect the spinal cord to various parts of the body.

As the spinal cord approaches the tail bone (coccyx) it forms separate nerves that collectively are known as the cauda equina (Latin for horse's tail). These nerves supply the hips, legs, ankles, feet and toes.

Spinal joints

Between every two vertebrae are joints formed by smooth cartilage and strengthened by ligaments that run behind and in front of the vertebral bodies throughout the entire length of the spine. In addition, there are facet joints at the back of the vertebrae.

The facets – so-called because of their smooth surface, like that of a cut gem – form joints (facet joints) with those of the vertebrae above and below. Each joint is surrounded by synovial membrane, which secretes a lubricating fluid (synovial fluid). The joint surfaces are covered with a smooth cartilage that facilitates the moving of one vertebra on the other.

Intervertebral discs

Between the weight-bearing part of adjacent vertebrae, from the second cervical to the sacrum, are intervertebral discs. Each disc consists of an outer fibrous ring (annulus fibrosus) and an inner substance that is soft and elastic (nucleus pulposus). The discs allow the spine a range of movement and absorb shock. When compressed they flatten, broaden and bulge.

Spinal ligaments

The spine is supported by strong fibres called ligaments. They hold the bones together and give strength to all the joints. In addition, they limit movement and so help to prevent damage.

Spinal tendons

Attaching muscles to the spinal bones are fibrous bands called tendons. When your back muscles contract, they pull on tendons, which then move your spine.

Interestingly, since both tendons and ligaments are subjected to a great deal of pulling, they do not have a very rich blood and nerve supply. They therefore depend on surrounding tissues for much of their oxygen and nutrients. This partly explains why they take a long time to heal when injured.

Sacrum and pelvis

At the juncture where the sacrum and coccyx meet the hip bones are the sacroiliac joints. They are part of the pelvis (pelvic ring or pelvic girdle).

The pelvic ring is the body's chief weight-transmitting structure, connecting its upper part to the legs. One of its key characteristics is that the degree of its tilt affects the normal spinal curves. An abnormal tilt of the pelvic ring contributes to poor posture, which can render the spine more vulnerable to injury and pain than a normally balanced pelvis.

Supporting muscles

Giving support and strength to the spine are various muscles, essentially those of the back and, indirectly, those of the abdomen and legs. Below is a brief description of the major supporting muscles.

The back

The erector spinae form two columns, one on each side of the spine. They keep the trunk erect. They also extend the spine, control forwards bending (flexion), sideward bending and rotation.

The latissimus dorsi is a broad, flat muscle that lies over the lower part of the chest and loins. It draws the upper arm bone down and back and rotates the arm inwards.

The gluteus maximus forms the buttocks. It raises the trunk from a stooping to an upright position. It is also involved in leg movements such as walking, running and jumping.

The trapezius runs from the back of the neck and along the shoulders. It draws the head back and the shoulders together and so expands the chest.

The abdomen

Weak abdominal muscles commonly contribute to backache, because they work in collaboration with the back muscles, providing spinal reinforcement. The following four sets form an 'abdominal corset':

The rectus abdominis is a long, flat muscle that runs along the front of the abdomen, from the breastbone to the pubic bones, on each side of an imaginary line down the middle. It flexes the spine (as when bending forwards) and it supports the abdominal organs.

The obliquus externus abdominis, with fibres running obliquely from the lower ribs to the pelvis (at the crest of the hip), rotates the trunk and flexes it sideways. It also gives support to organs within the trunk.

The obliquus internus abdominis occupies the same location as the obliquus externus muscles, but its fibres run in the opposite direction. The two work together to produce the same actions.

The transversalis abdominis lies beneath the two sets of oblique muscles and assists them in their functions.

Further reinforcing the back muscles is a fifth set of abdominals – the **quadratus lumborum**. They lie in the lumbar region on each side of the spine and run from the last rib to the iliac crest of the hip. They assist the other abdominal muscles.

The legs

Certain leg muscles are regarded as secondary back supports. Two of these, the quadriceps and the hamstrings, contribute to the balance of the pelvic ring and so help to maintain normal spinal curves and, consequently, good posture.

The psoas muscle passes along the groin and inserts into the upper thigh bone. The iliacus arises from the hip bone and unites with the psoas. The two together, called the ilio-psoas, flex and rotate the thighs (hip flexors).

The quadriceps, four in number, are located on the front of the thighs. They arise from the pelvic and thigh bones and insert into the upper knee cap. They extend, or straighten, the knees.

The hamstrings (also called the semitendinosus), of which there are three on each leg, run along the back of the thighs. They pass from the pelvis and insert into the lower leg bones. They flex the legs and move them towards the middle of the body (adduct them). They also extend the thighs.

The gluteal muscles tighten the thighs and move them away from the body (abduct them).

Understanding how the spine is constructed and how it functions helps us to appreciate why certain back problems occur. It can give us insight into how to take care of our backs and so prevent some difficulties from arising.

What Can Go Wrong

When you consider how intricate the construction of the spine is and how varied are its components, you can readily understand why neck and back problems are so common and widespread.

This chapter examines what can go wrong with each of the parts that make up the spine and its related structures and gives examples of conditions that can occur because of departures from normal functioning. These disorders are discussed in detail in the chapter on ailments (page 114), in which treatment options are also suggested.

Back and neck pain

Not all back and neck pain is experienced as a result of an injury or repetitive strain. Pain can occur as a result of a problem elsewhere in the body, such as a bladder infection, stomach ulcer or even psychological complications.

Spinal pain

Back and neck pain can occur because of biomechanical problems such as compression of intervertebral discs, torsion (twisting) injury and vibration, such as that produced by some types of tools (jackhammers, for example). People whose occupations require strenuous or repetitive lifting in a stooped position are most at risk of experiencing these difficulties.

Spinal pain can also be a result of destructive forces that occur in infections, tumours and rheumatoid disorders such as arthritis and ankylosing spondylitis (page 122).

Degenerative changes, as seen in osteoporosis and spinal stenosis (narrowed spinal canal), are other sources of back and neck pain. Because osteoporotic bones are not as strong as healthy ones, they are more vulnerable to collapse, causing pressure on nerves, which in turn may produce pain. In spinal stenosis, the narrowing of the canal through which the spinal cord runs, and consequent compression of nerves, is what generates pain.

Non-spinal back pain

Back and neck pain can be associated with a number of health disorders not originating in the spine. These include:

Stomach or duodenal ulcer

Inflammation of the pancreas (pancreatitis)

Enlarged abdominal aorta (large artery)

Bladder or kidney infection

Gynaecological conditions such as fibroids, endometriosis, dysmenorrhoea and pelvic infection

Pregnancy-related problems including ectopic pregnancy (occurring in an abnormal position)

Psychogenic pain

Pain originating from psychological sources, such as depression, a significant personal loss or other life crisis, is yet another cause of spinal problems. This may be explained, in part, by the way the brain processes pain and by the suppression of endorphins, which are the body's own pain-relievers.

Red flags

Of all the conditions that can trigger neck and back pain, there are some that signal serious health disorders. They are therefore called 'red flags' and they require urgent medical attention. They include:

Recent major trauma such as injury from a car accident or sports event

Pain that worsens at night or when you lie down

Fever which cannot be explained

Weight loss or gain which cannot be explained

A history of cancer, diabetes, kidney disease or osteoporosis

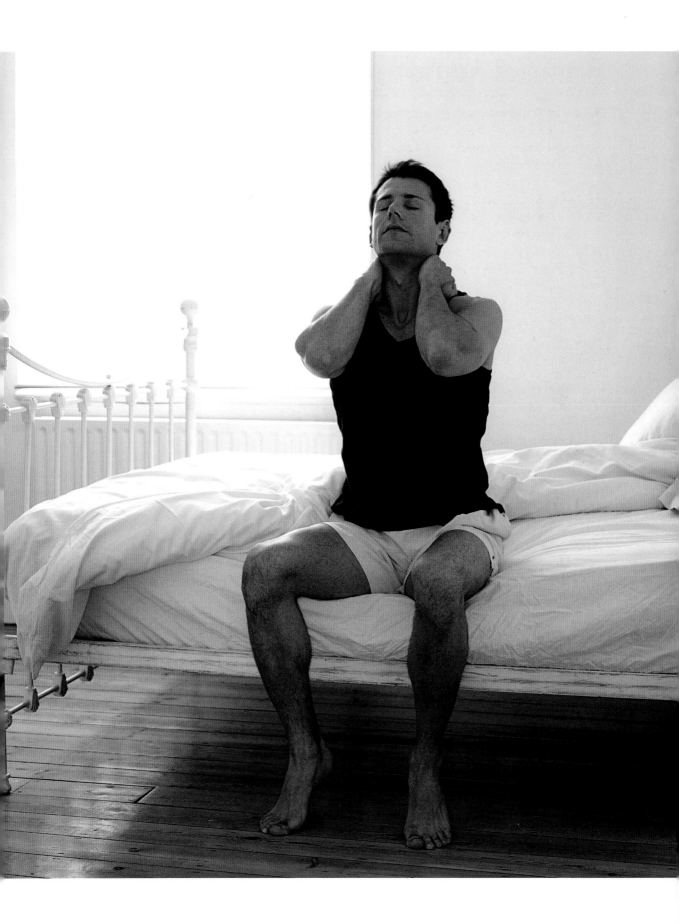

Spinal components

Below is a list of the various parts that make up the spine and examples of what can go wrong with each of them. Later in the chapter, we look at diagnostic procedures that help to identify specific disorders.

SPINAL CORD AND NERVES
Spinal cord damage
Irritation (of the sciatic nerve, for example) leading to sciatica
Inflammation
Compression of nerves
Impingement on nerves
(as in spinal stenosis)
Cauda equina syndrome

DISCS
Herniation
(as may occur in the cervical vertebrae in whiplash)
Degeneration
Strain

TENDONS
Tendons are vulnerable to the same injuries as ligaments (below left).

BONES
Bruises
Fractures
Trauma (as from a fall)
Loss of bone mass
(as in osteoporosis)
Infection
Malignancy

ABNORMAL SPINAL CURVES
Scoliosis
(lateral spinal curvature)
Lordosis
(abnormal forward curve of the lumbar spine)
Kyphosis
(posterior curvature of the thoracic spine; hump-back, as is sometimes seen in osteoarthritis)

MUSCLES
Muscle spasm
(as sometimes occurs in whiplash)
Strain
Tears
Tightness
Inflammation
Overuse

JOINTS
Degenerative changes
(as in osteoarthritis)
Strain
Slippage
(as in spondylolisthesis)
Cumulative stress
Poor posture
Swelling
Strain or arthritis of the facet joints

LIGAMENTS
Tears
Strain
Sprain
Trauma
(as may be sustained in a sports accident)
Cumulative stress
(repetitive strain)
Pregnancy-related
(lax sacroiliac ligaments, due to hormonal influence)

MULTIPLE STRUCTURES
The following conditions can affect various spinal structures:
Whiplash
Degenerative changes
Inflammation
Instability
(such as the slippage that occurs in spondylolisthesis)

Diagnostic tests

In order to identify the cause and nature of your back and neck pain and associated symptoms, your doctor may order one or more of a number of tests. These are used to confirm a diagnosis based on a physical examination. They may also be done to rule out certain other suspected disorders, or as part of preparation for surgery. In addition, they are useful in helping to plan treatment. The following are some of the more common procedures in current use.

MRI scan
(Magnetic Resonance Imaging)

Instead of X-rays, this test uses changing magnetic fields to provide images of various body structures. Tissues in different parts have different resonance properties. Changes in these properties occur in disease states such as inflammation. MRI scans are useful in their detection.

MRI provides an excellent picture of the spine and also of soft tissues such as discs, muscles and ligaments. It is therefore very useful for evaluating conditions such as a narrowed spinal canal (spinal stenosis), spinal cord damage, infection and tumours. It is also of value when surgery is being contemplated for spinal stenosis and some cases of disc herniation.

The procedure requires you to lie very still for perhaps an hour, in a small tube, and you will be screened in advance for the presence of any metallic device or objects in your body. People with claustrophobia may be given anxiety-relieving medication.

MRI MAY BE ORDERED FOR
- Emergency evaluation of Cauda Equina Syndrome (page 117)
- Progressive neurologic symptoms
- Symptoms suggesting infection or tumour
- Evaluation of spinal stenosis pre-operatively
- Evaluation of disc herniation pre-operatively
- Evaluation of degenerative changes in recurring or persisting back pain

MRI IS NOT ADVISED
- In pregnancy
- Following recent blood vessel surgery
- In severe claustrophobia
- In the presence of a heart pacemaker or metal objects in the body

Plain X-rays
(radiographs)

Plain X-rays of the spine show the spinal column, sacrum and sacroiliac joints. They are useful in assessing bone quality and revealing arthritic changes and narrowed disc spaces. Your doctor will probably order a plain X-ray in the following instances:
- Red flag conditions (page 16)
- Severe injury and suspected fractures
- A history of osteoporosis or cancer
- Severe pain at night, which worsens or is unrelieved by rest

A plain X-ray may also be ordered if you report:
- Persisting back pain
- Symptoms suggesting unstable vertebrae ('catching')
- Suspected arthritic changes, such as pain and impaired function

X-rays are not advisable during pregnancy because of possible damage to the foetus.

CT scan
(Computerized Tomography)

Formerly called a CAT (Computerized Axial Tomography) scan, this procedure uses regular X-rays to provide a three-dimensional image of body structures. It is a painless procedure that requires the client to be on a platform that passes through a horseshoe-shaped gantry (special supporting structure).

The CT scan provides good visualisation of bony structures and also of soft tissues such as nerves, discs and ligaments. It is therefore useful in identifying conditions such as spinal stenosis, disc herniation and nerve compression and bone erosions due to infection or tumour. It is also of value in the pre-operative assessment of some conditions, such as spinal stenosis due to arthritis.

Post-operatively, a CT scan helps the surgeon to assess correct placement following the implantation of hardware such as screws and plates – in spinal fusion, for example.

Although exposure to radiation is minimal, a CT scan should be used with caution, if at all, on pregnant women.

Isotope bone scan
(Technetium and SPECT)

This test measures bone cell activity. It requires the injection of a harmless radioactive marker into a vein in the hand, followed two hours later by a scan of the whole body or a specific part. Active areas show up as 'hot spots'.

This bone scan is very sensitive in detecting fractures and it can pick up minor bone injuries not visible on X-rays. It can help to distinguish an acute fracture from an old one. It is also a sensitive test for the presence of infection and tumour metastases. It can, in addition, reveal the presence of osteoporosis.

As with other tests that involve radiation, the isotope bone scan is not advised during pregnancy.

Myelography

Myelography requires the injection of a radiopaque dye into the sheath containing the spinal cord and nerve roots. The dye facilitates imaging. Plain X-rays are then taken. The procedure is useful in assessing conditions such as nerve compression and spinal cord abnormalities.

Myelography necessitates the insertion of a long needle into the back, and its side effects include headache and nerve irritation. Although it is sometimes used in conjunction with a CT scan, it has largely been replaced by MRI (page 19).

SPECT scan (Single-Proton Emission Computerized Tomography)

A SPECT scan works in a similar way to a regular bone scan, and like a CT scan it can give three-dimensional localisation. This has proven particularly useful in identifying arthritic facet joints prior to injection therapy, and for post-operative evaluation of spinal fusion.

The SPECT scan does not replace a CT scan or an MRI, but it may be useful in acquiring more information about the precise location of a problem.

Discography

Discography requires the insertion of a needle into an intervertebral disc, with the help of X-ray guidance. This is followed by the injection of radiopaque dye and saline (salt water).

Discography is useful in the assessment of disc integrity and is usually performed without sedation or general anaesthesia because the patient must be sufficiently alert to report what he or she is feeling. Local anaesthetic, however, can be used on the skin prior to needle insertion.

Uses for discography include:

* Identifying the intervertebral disc as a cause of low back pain
* As an aid in predicting the probable outcome of certain invasive disc procedures
* As an aid in planning surgery and predicting its probable outcome

Blood tests

The following are some tests that may be ordered to help identify the source of neck and back pain (see also Glossary, page 136):

* CBC (complete blood count) and ESR (erythrocyte sedimentation rate) in the presence of red flag conditions (page 16), or when pain persists for several weeks
* CBC, ESR, C-reactive protein, TB test and blood cultures to help detect possible infection
* CBC, ESR, calcium phosphate, serum protein levels and analysis, liver enzymes, PSA (prostate gland screen) in men, to help detect possible malignancy
* CBC, ESR, rheumatology screen and HLA-B27 screen to help detect spinal pathology such as arthritis and ankylosing spondylitis

Nerve tests

Certain nerve tests may be carried out either for purposes of diagnosis or for monitoring during major spinal surgery. They include:

* EMG (electromyography) to test the function of motor nerves, which enable muscles to contract
* SSEPs (somatosensory evoked potentials), which test the integrity of sensory nerves
* Nerve conduction tests, which examine the transmission speed of electrical impulses along a nerve

Coping With Pain

Pain is more than just an unpleasant sensory and emotional experience. It is whatever and wherever the person feeling it says it is. He or she is the only one who can most accurately describe it.

Functions of pain

Pain is a warning signal to alert us to possible harm. As such, it is a protective mechanism, the essential value of which is that of survival. Pain also serves as a basis for learning and helps us to avoid potentially injurious objects and situations. In addition, pain arising from already damaged tissues helps to promote recovery: it does this by limiting activity and enforcing the rest and relaxation necessary for recuperation and healing.

Pain perception

Because the perception and interpretation of pain are based on individual experience, they are different for everyone. How we perceive and interpret pain depends not only on the degree of physical damage, but also on other factors such as anxiety, depression, attention, expectation, tolerance, past experience and cultural learning.

Pain pathway

The network that relays impulses and sensations related to disease or trauma may be thought of as a pain pathway. The 'gate control' theory of pain was first put forward by the Canadian psychologist Ronald Melzack and the British physiologist Patrick Wall in the 1960s. It attempted to explain how this pathway works. Since it provides some basis for why certain pain-relieving techniques work (such as acupuncture, massage and TENS, which we look at later in the book), it will be described briefly.

'Gate control'

Melzack and Wall proposed the existence of a nervous system mechanism that, in effect, opens or closes a 'gate' to increase or decrease the flow of nerve impulses to the brain. This mechanism can be influenced by certain psychological factors (page 34), and partly explains why some people tolerate pain better than others.

Some natural pain-control methods (yoga techniques, for example) are largely based on closing this spinal gate to prevent noxious stimuli from reaching the brain. These practices are essentially based on the concept that certain signals can be blocked at the earliest stages of nervous system transmission. They mobilise the body's own resources for promoting pain relief and healing.

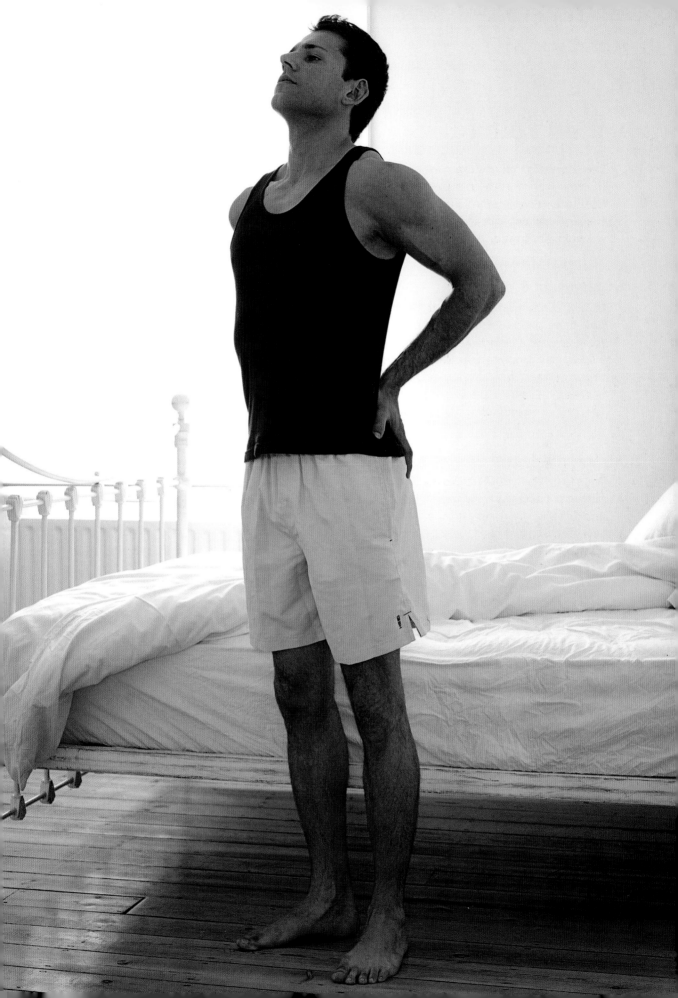

Pain relief

The choices for relief from back and neck pain are numerous. Pain-relief measures can be non-invasive, such as local applications of cold and heat, or invasive, such as injected medications or surgery. All aim to ease discomfort and suffering, improve mobility, restore function and enhance the quality of life. The three main types of pain you might experience – acute pain, chronic pain or referred pain – are explained below.

Acute pain

Usually lasts less than six months, tends to have an identifiable onset. Its duration is often predictable and it generally disappears as the condition that produces it resolves. This type of pain is frequently described as 'sharp' or 'shooting'. It is usually reversible, or controllable with adequate treatment.

Chronic pain

Tends to be slow in onset and to vary in intensity from mild to severe. It is constant or recurring and generally has no predictable end. It usually lasts more than six months. Because chronic pain syndromes are often described in vague terms, and because many of their causes are difficult to identify, their treatments can be diverse. Chronic pain may be divided into three types:

Chronic non-malignant pain, as from a low back disorder, rheumatoid arthritis or whiplash.

Chronic intermittent pain, as from some form of arthritis.

Chronic malignant pain, as from cancer.

Because of its prolonged nature, chronic pain tends to be more difficult to bear than pain of short duration. It often generates mood and behavioural changes, which include anxiety, depression, sleeplessness, fatigue and an increase or decrease of appetite with consequent weight gain or loss.

Referred pain

Is felt at a site different from that of the injured or diseased body part. An example is pain from gall bladder disease, which may be felt in the upper back near the right shoulder blade.

Physical therapies

Your choice of pain relief therapy will largely depend on your specific problem and also on your ability to tolerate pain and associated symptoms (see page 24). Physical therapies represent an important choice of pain relief therapy for many back and neck conditions. Often, they may be all that is needed to alleviate pain and restore function.

Cryotherapy

The application of cold (cryotherapy) in the treatment of acute pain has been used for centuries. Cold lowers the temperature of the skin and underlying tissues, decreases bleeding by constricting blood vessels and decreases muscle spasm and local tissue metabolism.

Perhaps the most efficient way to apply cold is to put crushed ice in a plastic bag and wrap it in a damp towel. Apply it to the affected area for about 20 minutes during the first 48 to 72 hours of acute low back pain or lumbar strain. Allow approximately 40 minutes to elapse before reapplication.

You can also try a re-usable 'gel' pack, but, to avoid frostbite, be sure to wrap it in a thin towel and not apply it directly to the skin. Caution is advised in using cold applications if you suffer from rheumatoid arthritis.

Superficial heat therapy

Applying heat to a painful area reduces muscle spasm and promotes relaxation and comfort. It also increases tissue metabolism and blood flow, with a resulting decrease in pain.

In general, superficial heat is applied through heat packs or heating blankets. It is used after the first 48 to 72 hours of an episode of low back pain. It is also employed in some cases of chronic back pain and muscle spasm.

This form of heat should not be used during the initial inflammatory stages of conditions such as acute lumbar strain (which would be treated with ice for the first 48 to 72 hours, prior to applying heat).

Do not use heat if your back pain is due to an accident, such as a fall or a blow to your back.

Ultrasound

In ultrasound treatment, high-frequency sound waves are applied to affected tissues. To administer therapy, a trained practitioner uses a·hand-held probe attached to an ultrasound machine.

Ultrasound treatment is particularly useful for muscle and tendon injuries: it improves blood flow, eases muscle spasm and relieves pain. At lower levels, ultrasound may also be used to promote the healing of fractures and the repair of cartilage. The use of ultrasound is not advised:

In some arthritic conditions, in which heat may actually speed up joint deterioration.

In the presence of certain inflammatory conditions or blood disorders.

Over tumours, whether they are malignant or not

For pain relief during pregnancy.

Short-wave diathermy

Similar in effect to ultrasound, short-wave diathermy involves the passage of a high-frequency current to create a rapid vibration that provides deep heat to tissues.

As with other deep-heat treatments, short-wave diathermy should not be used in the acute phases of low back pain, nor should it be used near metal implants or if you have a heart pacemaker.

Hydrotherapy

The external use of water-based treatments is known as hydrotherapy. It takes advantage of the therapeutic properties of water: cold to constrict surface blood vessels and limit inflammation; hot to dilate blood vessels, increase blood flow and induce relaxation. Improved circulation facilitates the delivery of oxygen and nutrients to tissues and the removal of body wastes. It also boosts the immune system and promotes healing.

Some therapies use cold and hot water alternately. This is believed to stimulate the endocrine (hormonal) system, reduce congestion and relieve inflammation.

When you exercise in water, unimpeded by gravity, your spine is not subjected to strain, and so this therapy is of value to those who suffer from low back pain, for example. Many hospital physiotherapy departments have a hydrotherapy pool, which people with back complaints can use with supervision. In some European countries, hydrotherapy is one of the main treatments for back problems.

Hydrotherapy treatments also include whirl-pool baths, in which the body is immersed in pressurised bubbles for about 15 minutes. The water temperature can be regulated to suit individual requirements. However, to prevent even the slightest risk of infection, these baths are best avoided in the first fortnight following surgery.

Soaking in water with a temperature of about 38 degrees Celsius (100 degrees Fahrenheit) for 20 to 30 minutes is believed to help in relieving some arthritic conditions. Therapeutic oils and herbs can be added to the water.

TENS

(Transcutaneous Electrical Nerve Stimulation: trans = through; cutaneous = skin)
Also referred to as electrical nerve stimulation, TENS uses a low-voltage electrical current, applied to the skin, to stimulate nerves and muscles.

Although there is uncertainty as to how this procedure works, the belief is that it alters the body's ability to perceive and feel pain, in accord with the spinal gate theory (page 24).

TENS has been used mostly to relieve chronic and recurrent back pain, but it has also been useful for facilitating rehabilitation following sports injuries, and can be used in combination with other methods to relieve pain and restore function. The circumstances when TENS should not be used include:
During pregnancy.
In the presence of heart irregularities or a heart pacemaker.
For application to areas near the throat.
Where there is an infection or tumour.

Traction

Traction is the application of a pulling force to a body part while a countertraction pulls in the opposite direction. The pulling force can be achieved by using the hands (manual traction) or by the use of weights. For centuries, traction has been used as therapy for low back pain, using a pelvic sling, weights and pulleys.

The purposes of traction include:
Reducing, realigning and promoting the healing of fractured bones.
Decreasing muscle spasms that may accompany fractures or following surgery, or spasms associated with whiplash or low back pain.
Immobilising body parts to prevent soft tissue. damage.
Restoring inflamed, painful or diseased joints.
Relieving pressure on spinal nerves and intervertebral discs.
One disadvantage of traction is the possibility of prolonged bed rest (see page 129).

Gravity traction

This involves hanging upside down, using gravity boots or a similar inversion device, and aims at widening the spaces between vertebrae in order to relieve pressure on discs.

This is usually a physically demanding procedure, and is sometimes associated with headache and increased blood pressure and heart rate. It should, therefore, be avoided if you have hypertension or glaucoma.

Braces and supports

Braces and back supports can be useful during the acute phase of certain types of back pain, or as a preventive measure for those who are prone to back problems and anticipate a physically demanding day. These devices help to support the back and maintain good posture. They include corsets and a variety of lumbar supports.

Beneficial as these can be, they nevertheless do some of the work that your own muscles should be doing. When muscles are not exercised regularly, they weaken and become more vulnerable to injury. The use of braces and supports should therefore be limited.

Orthotics

Your gait, which is your own special style of walking, affects your wellbeing much like posture does. This is because gait largely determines the distribution of stress on various parts of your feet and legs.

The type of footwear you use affects your gait. If your shoes fit poorly, they may force you to arch your spine too far forwards or backwards, for example, and so alter your posture. This may have a negative impact on your neck and back and may lead to strains, sprains and other disorders.

Orthotics are devices, such as inserts placed in footwear, to help improve your gait and, consequently, your posture and spinal health. They should not, by themselves, be considered as therapy for backache, but rather as part of a comprehensive treatment plan that involves other medical specialities.

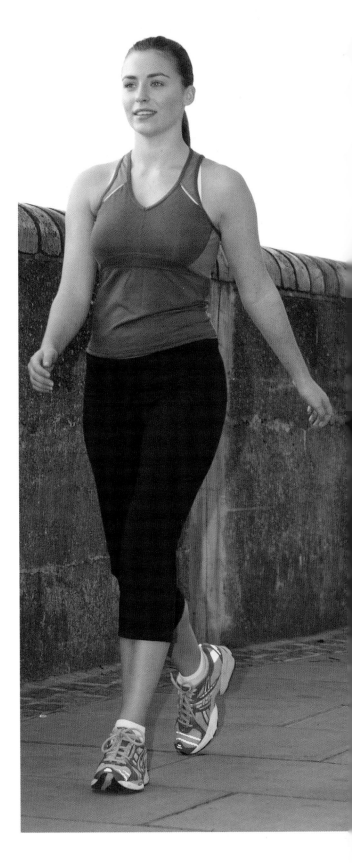

Hands-on therapies

The sense of touch, which is most closely associated with the skin (our largest organ), is the earliest to develop in the human embryo. Both skin and nervous system arise from the ectoderm, which is the general surface covering of the embryonic body. The skin may, therefore, be regarded as an exposed portion of the nervous system. It is also an important part of the immune system, which helps to protect us from agents of disease.

Benefits of touch

Hands-on therapies, which employ human touch, take advantage of the importance of the skin's tactile functions. The biochemical benefits of touching have been well documented – for example, babies who are frequently held and touched have fewer illnesses and thrive better than those who are not.

Massage

Massage therapy may be defined as the treatment of disease by manual manipulation. Although various hand-held electrical and non-electrical massage devices are available, there is no substitute for human hands.

One way in which massage is thought to bring pain relief is by blocking noxious stimuli (see 'spinal gate' theory, page 24). Another is by stimulating the release of the body's own pain relievers – endorphins and enkaphalins.

Massage can be beneficial in treating some cases of neck and low back pain and conditions associated with them, such as anxiety and sleeplessness and the stress inherent in chronic low back pain. Massage is employed for varied reasons including:

Relieving spasms and pain.
Inducing relaxation.
Stretching muscles and improving muscle tone.
Breaking down adhesions and scar tissue.
Increasing blood flow, metabolism and the elimination of wastes.
Enhancing mobility.
Beneficial as massage can be, it should not be performed:
Over or close to an ulcerated lesion or cancerous tumour.

Over the sacral area in the first eight months of pregnancy.
When back pain is due to a fall or other injury.

Shiatsu

The art of Shiatsu – a Japanese word that literally means 'finger pressure' – is based on Traditional Chinese Medicine and on Western anatomy and physiology. Its principles are very similar to those of acupuncture (page 30) but without the use of needles.

Shiatsu has been proven effective in decreasing the level of anxiety associated with continual back pain. It is usually employed as part of a more comprehensive treatment plan for the relief of certain back disorders and some forms of arthritis.

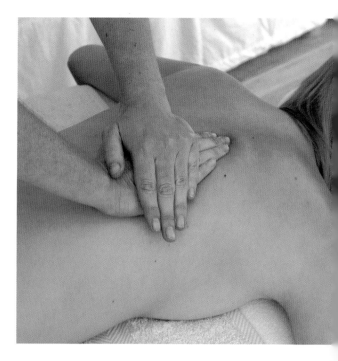

Acupressure

Part of Traditional Chinese Medicine and sometimes referred to as 'acupuncture without needles', acupressure involves the application of pressure, using fingers and thumbs, to stimulate and regulate the body's healing energy (chi or qi).

It is based on the belief that healing energy circulates throughout the body along specific pathways called meridians, and that disease is a result of blockages in this energy current. Acupressure is believed to release these obstructions through the application of pressure on certain points (acupoints) along the meridians.

Conditions that can respond favourably to acupressure include some types of neck, shoulder and back pain, sciatica (page 116) and rheumatism.

Acupuncture

Based on the same principles as acupressure (see above), acupuncture involves the insertion of needles rather than the use of finger pressure. The needles are solid and very thin, and there is virtually no pain when they are inserted.

One way in which this therapy is believed to work is through the 'spinal gate' mechanism (page 24). It has been found beneficial in the relief of back pain, both acute and chronic, and in conditions such as sciatica. Its use is best avoided in pregnancy, however, since it may stimulate uterine contractions.

Reflexology

According to practitioners of reflexology, the feet and hands mirror the body. Pressure applied to them, at specific points, can affect corresponding areas of the body by stimulating natural healing powers.

The feet contain thousands of nerve endings. Pressure applied on them, through reflexology, can induce deep relaxation. It can facilitate free blood flow by which all tissues receive oxygen and nutrients.

Some types of back pain and associated conditions such as anxiety and other forms of stress have been relieved by reflexology.

Chiropractic

A widely practised branch of Western complementary medicine, chiropractic (from two Greek words: *cheior*, which means hand, and *praktikos*, which means doing) was developed in the late 1800s by a Canadian osteopath named Daniel David Palmer. Its aim is to diagnose and treat disorders of the spine, joints and muscles and to maintain the health of the central nervous system.

The key principle in chiropractic is based on the belief that any distortion of the spine, which links the body and the brain, will affect other parts of the anatomy. Chiropractors believe that when the skeletal structure is functioning smoothly, the body's natural healing forces will help the whole system to work harmoniously.

Chiropractic utilises essentially two types of manual manipulations to correct misalignments believed to be responsible for many cases of low back pain. Pain relief is believed to be brought about, in part, by a release of endorphins (the body's natural pain relievers).

Chiropractic treatments have been found useful in various conditions including some neck and back problems and some muscular, joint and postural conditions.

Although generally very safe, chiropractic is contraindicated in a number of disorders, which include nerve pain with numbness, cancer and severe osteoporosis.

Osteopathy

The practice of osteopathy was developed in the 1870s by an army doctor named Andrew Taylor Still. The therapy is based on the belief that the body will heal itself if given the right conditions.

Osteopathic manipulation aims to restore the flow of blood and lymph and the normal transmission of nerve impulses. Gentle pressure is applied predominantly to soft tissues rather than bones and joints. Manual therapy is sometimes combined with medications.

Osteopathy is a useful treatment option in some cases of uncomplicated neck and back pain, arthritic conditions, repetitive strain and sports injuries.

Posture and movement therapies

Posture generally refers to the position of your body in space. Body mechanics is the way you use your body and its parts in everyday activities. Both are important to health and wellbeing. They determine how much stress is placed on bones, muscles, tendons, spinal discs and other structures.

Good posture and body mechanics keep stress to a minimum and place it mostly on those structures that are best able to bear them. By contrast, poor habits of posture and movement can put the neck and rest of the spine at risk of strains, unnecessary pressure on nerves and other disorders, with resulting pain and dysfunction.

The posture and movement therapies that follow are among the most common in current practice. Their chief aims are to train subjects in the safest and most efficient use of their body and its parts in day-to-day living, and so help to prevent or alleviate pain and loss of function.

The Alexander Technique

This system of postural re-education was devised in the 1800s by an Australian actor named Frederick Matthias Alexander. Discouraged by medical treatments that could give him no more than temporary relief from a persisting hoarseness that affected his acting, Alexander set about finding a more satisfactory solution. He found that by improving postural patterns and body mechanics, he could function more efficiently, with fewer instances of muscle tightness and pain.

The Alexander Technique focuses on changing improper ways of using the body and its parts in everyday activities, and encourages more efficient movement with minimal tension and effort and less stress on joints, muscles and related structures. This helps to prevent further injury and promote healing.

Best learned under the guidance of a teacher specially trained in the method, the Alexander Technique is useful for relieving some symptoms of whiplash, back pain, repetitive strain injury, sciatica and rheumatism, and conditions associated with these disorders, such as anxiety.

The Feldenkrais Method

Named after Dr Moshe Feldenkrais, this physical re-education system was developed in the 1940s. Its aims are to explore body awareness and improve flexibility and range of motion.

The method is based on the belief that habitual faulty postures and body movements disrupt the nervous system, and identifying and correcting these disruptions helps to restore normal functioning. The method also employs 'functional integration', which uses touch and manipulation tailored to individual needs.

The Feldenkrais Method may be considered a useful treatment option in some cases of spinal and muscular pain and in some sports injuries.

The Rosen Method

Devised in the 1940s by physiotherapist Marion Rosen, this system of emotional and physical therapy aims at restoring the natural balance that is characteristic of a healthy mind and body. It attempts to do this by releasing tensions and blockages and correcting unhealthy behaviours. It also recognises the role of emotions in physical wellbeing and the link between breathing and feelings. Accordingly, the method avails itself of various techniques including posture education and massage, and flexibility, breathing and relaxation exercises.

The Rosen Method is a worthwhile option to explore, particularly by those who have chronic back pain and associated stresses, and where other therapies have failed.

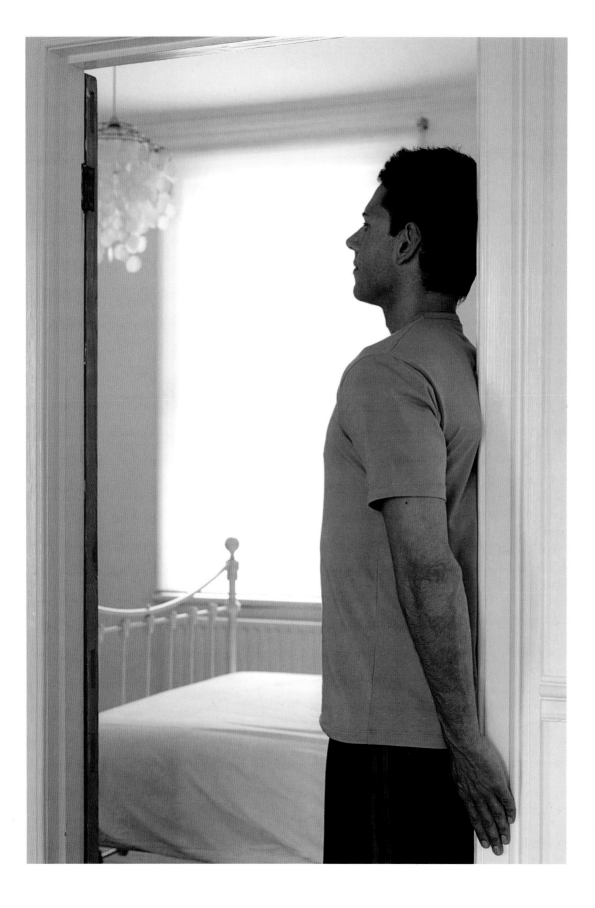

Mind-body therapies

The 'gate control' theory of pain (page 24) suggests that some pain-relieving techniques, such as imagery and visualisation or hypnotheraphy, can help to prevent messages of pain from reaching the brain. The following are just a few of the psychological methods that help to decrease pain from unbearable to bearable levels, promote a sense of self-control and decrease feelings of powerlessness. They utilise techniques that include suggestion, distraction and relaxation.

Autogenic Training

Developed in the 1900s by a German physician named Johannes Schultz, Autogenic Training is a type of relaxation technique. It consists of the mental repetition of verbal phrases, such as 'my right arm is heavy', intended to improve muscular relaxation and blood flow and is an organised way of helping to counteract stress and mobilise the body's self-healing resources.

Autogenic Training is a useful treatment option to consider in conditions where pain may be attributed to, or aggravated by, stress.

Biofeedback

Biofeedback uses electronic monitoring devices, connected by electrodes to the skin, to gather information on body functions such as muscle contractions, heart rate and brain wave activity. This information is 'fed back' to the person undergoing the therapy, who is then taught appropriate relaxation techniques. By practising these exercises, the person learns to gain a measure of control over certain body responses formerly believed to be entirely involuntary, such as blood flow and skin temperature. Biofeedback has been found particularly useful in some chronic pain states and in stress-related conditions.

Cognitive Behavioural Therapy

This is a form of psychotherapy that aims to alter negative thought patterns and attitudes in order to change behaviour.

Studies indicate that more than 50 per cent of patients reporting unpleasant physical symptoms that have no traceable underlying physical cause, nevertheless suffer from anxiety or depression. These patients, it was found, tended to indulge in negative emotions and behaviours that exacerbated their symptoms. For such patients, Cognitive Behavioural Therapy may be a worthwhile alternative to medication. Treatment options include relaxation training, cognitive restructuring techniques and role-playing exercises.

Hypnotherapy

Modern hypnotherapy evolved from the work of the Austrian physician Franz Anton Mesmer, from whose name the word 'mesmerise' originates.

Practitioners of this therapy induce in their subjects an altered state of consciousness that renders them receptive to suggestion. Individuals vary in their susceptibility to hypnosis, but an estimated 90 per cent of people can be hypnotised.

Conditions most amenable to hypnotherapy include anxiety and acute pain. It may also be used to decrease the need for medication.

Imagery and Visualisation

Imagery is a flow of thoughts and includes qualities from one or more of the senses. It has been used successfully in many mind-body therapies, including Autogenic Training, biofeedback and hypnosis. Imagery has also been employed in preparing patients for medical procedures and for the relief of pain and anxiety. It can, in addition, help to reduce the need for medications, and it has been found useful in the management of chronic arthritic pain, to relax muscles and decrease sensitivity to pain.

Visualisation is a technique that uses the imagination in a purposeful way to form mental pictures. Some people have been able to cope with physical and emotional problems by visualising positive images and desired outcomes, either by themselves or with the help of a practitioner.

Like imagery, visualisation is part of many relaxation therapies and is sometimes used as an adjunct to conventional cancer treatments. Its main uses include allaying anxiety and relieving pain and stress-related conditions.

Although the mechanisms underlying imagery and visualisations are not fully understood, the belief is that harnessing the powers of the imagination affects certain mental processes that facilitate coping with various dysfunctions.

Progressive Relaxation

Relaxation is said to be the common denominator of all therapies for relieving pain. It is also an essential prerequisite for healing any disorder.

One of the most effective and widely practised relaxation techniques is a method called Progressive Relaxation, the developing of which, in the 1930s, has been attributed to the American physiologist Dr Edmund Jacobson. In reality, however, this technique has been used by yoga practitioners for at least two thousand years – it is known as Savasana.

Progressive Relaxation involves the conscious contracting of muscle groups followed by releasing the contraction, so as to experience and compare the difference between tense and relaxed states. This is done in a systematic and progressive way until the whole body has attained deep relaxation.

The exercise decreases sympathetic nervous system responses, as occur when preparing for 'fight or flight', and increases parasympathetic nervous system activity, which induces a state of calm. Its main uses include the relief of anxiety and pain, but it may also be used as an adjunct to other treatments to enhance their effectiveness.

Relaxation Response

The relaxation response is elicited to counteract the 'fight or flight' response to stress. It reduces sympathetic nervous system activity and produces a calming effect. It is, therefore, a useful antidote to states such as anxiety, which intensify pain. Four essential components are required to elicit the relaxation response. They are:

A comfortable body position that enables you to be still for five to twenty minutes

Quiet surroundings and no interruptions

A slow and even breathing pattern

The repetition of a word or short phrase on every exhalation to keep you focused.

Voluntary Controlled Respiration

An unmistakable link exists between your breathing and your emotional state. When you are anxious, for instance, your breathing will probably be fast, and when you are in pain it will perhaps be shallow and sometimes irregular.

You can, however, influence your emotional state to some extent by wilfully altering your breathing pattern. You can do this because your respiratory (breathing) system is not only involuntary, but to some degree voluntary, also. By practising voluntary controlled respiration, you can actively contribute to the effectiveness of any treatment that aims at coping with stress and managing pain.

Most mind-body therapies (pages 34) employ exercises in voluntary controlled breathing to help achieve their goals. Many of them also combine breathing with visualisation for enhanced effects.

T'ai Chi Ch'uan

This non-combative martial art employs sequences of slow, graceful movements and breathing techniques to improve the flow of life energy, chi or qi (page 30), and so promote healing. It is, in effect, a type of mind-body practice that fosters improved musculoskeletal functioning.

T'ai Chi has been found to help relax the muscular and nervous systems, improve posture and flexibility and relieve symptoms of stress. It has long been used therapeutically among the elderly to help decrease pain perception and anxiety and improve balance, to lessen the risk of falls and injury. Other benefits reported have included the management of pain from ankylosing spondylitis (page 122).

Yoga

This centuries-old system aims at maintaining wellness of body, mind and spirit and restoring it when health has been disrupted. As practised by millions worldwide, it essentially comprises non-strenuous stretching and strengthening exercises, the practise of conscious breathing, exercises in balance, coordination, meditation and relaxation, and simple hygiene practices. It now forms the basis of many stress management, health promotion and childbirth education programmes.

Yoga is worthy of consideration as an adjunct to other therapies for relieving pain, improving balance, coordination and relaxation and promoting healing.

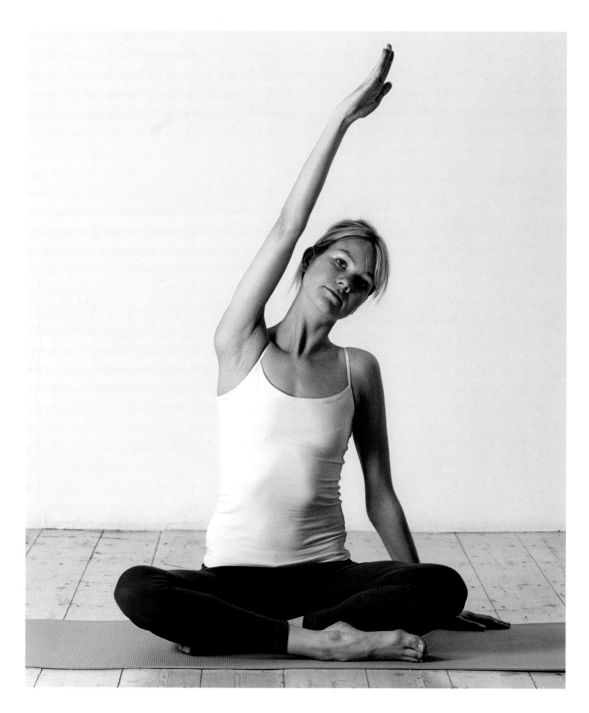

Medications

Medicines used to relieve pain and its attendant symptoms are numerous. They can be administered in various ways: by mouth (orally), by insertion into the rectum (rectally), by placing under the tongue (sublingually), by inhalation, or by injection into the tissues. Some can also be injected into the spinal canal or into selected nerves to produce nerve blocks.

Non-narcotics

This group of pain-relievers (analgesics) includes: aspirin, NSAIDs (non-steroidal anti-inflammatory drugs; pronounced 'en-seds') and paracetamol (a pain-relieving medicine without the anti-inflammatory properties of aspirin). Except for paracetamol, they act primarily at the peripheral nervous system level, where they serve an anti-inflammatory function.

The main side effect reported from NSAIDs is stomach irritation, which can lead to peptic ulcer and, particularly with aspirin, an increased tendency to bleed.

Narcotics (opoids)

These analgesics are all chemically related to morphine, which is extracted from poppies or other plants, or produced in a laboratory. They are usually used as part of a medication regimen when pain is moderate to severe. They work primarily at the central nervous system (CNS) level. Included in this group are morphine, pethidine (meperidine) and codeine.

The most bothersome side effects reported from using opoid analgesics are: constipation, nausea, and altered mental functioning, which makes tasks like driving and operating machinery inadvisable.

Adjuvant (assisting) analgesics

Adjuvant analgesics are drugs that are usually administered for purposes other than pain relief, but which nevertheless may have analgesic effects in some cases. They work in various ways and include: anticonvulsant (anti-seizure) agents such as phenytoin; antidepressants such as amitriptyline (which are sometimes useful in treating chronic low back pain), and muscle relaxants such as cyclobenzaprine. They may be used alone or combined with other medicines.

Nerve blocks

A nerve block is done by injecting a local anaesthetic around a nerve root as it exits the spinal canal. This inhibits nerve conduction to and from the area supplied by the nerve and weakens pain perception.

Sometimes a steroid is added to the local anaesthetic to reduce inflammation and swelling and to help promote the natural healing process. The procedure is often done in a series of three injections, with or without X-ray guidance to help with the correct placement of the needle. The more common sites for injection are the cervical and lumbar regions of the spine.

One of the most appropriate uses of this type of analgesia is for spinal stenosis (page 116), but it has also been found useful in other cases of low back pain and pain that radiates to the legs, to improve function and so enable the patient to participate in other therapies.

Chemonucleolysis

Chemonucleolysis is a less invasive alternative to surgery for patients between the ages of 18 and 50 years with symptoms of disc herniation.

The method (which is more popular in Europe than in America) requires the introduction of an enzyme called chymopapain (derived from the papaya plant) into the intervertebral disc, by way of a needle and X-ray guidance. The aim is to dissolve the inner disc core (nucleus pulposus, see page 12) and so reduce the herniation and its pressure on the nerve.

Among the conditions for which chemonucleolysis may be recommended are:
Leg pain, similar to that produced by sciatica.
Pain in raising the leg straight.
Ineffectiveness of more conservative treatments.
Desire to avoid surgery.

Caution
People who are planning to have this procedure done should first be tested for possible allergy to papaya. Pregnant women and people with a spinal tumour or neurological disorder such as multiple sclerosis should not undergo chemonucleolysis.

Combined therapies
Medication is often much more effective when combined with other forms of therapy, such as massage, progressive relaxation and visualisation. These and other similar treatments also sometimes help to reduce the dosage requirements of a particular medicine.

Surgical approaches

Estimates are that only two to five per cent of people with back pain and associated symptoms benefit from surgery. Even so, no back operation can guarantee desired results. But although surgery has limitations, it is never used as a last resort. Not smoking and not being overweight increase the chances of a successful outcome in all surgeries.

Decompression is one of the four categories of surgical procedure that might be employed. It removes pressure that causes symptoms such as back and leg pain, numbness and weakness. Discectomy, micro-discectomy and decompression are examples of this type of surgery.

The next category of procedure is stabilisation, which combines decompression with a procedure called 'fusion'. Restoring stability is usually achieved through the use of a bone graft and rods and screws inserted into the bone. This type of surgery may be done in fractures or where degenerative changes have put the spine's stability at risk.

Strengthening, through the injection of bone cement, is the third option. This is known as vertebroplasty. It is done to strengthen the bones, relieve pain and improve mobility following the collapse of a vertebra, as may occur in osteoporosis.

Finally, straightening can be used to remedy spinal deformity, such as that resulting from childhood scoliosis or adult disorders such as degenerative changes, infection and tumour. An example of this type of surgery, which also involves strengthening, is kyphoplasty (see kyphosis, page 127).

Discectomy
In this procedure, the centre of the disc (nucleus pulposus) is excised, or a laser is used to destroy damaged disc material. This type of surgery is usually reserved for people who have a disc herniation that produces persisting, severe, disabling leg symptoms.

Micro-discectomy
Probably the most successful method in current use for removing damaged disc material, this procedure employs micro-surgical instruments to remove fragments of a herniated (or ruptured) disc. Compared with standard surgery, this technique preserves more tissue integrity and causes less trauma. But although the procedure takes pressure off the affected nerve and improves day-to-day functioning, it does not completely eradicate the pain.

Decompression
This operation is usually done to treat spinal stenosis (page 116). Formerly, a great deal of bone

was removed from around the nerve root, resulting in some cases of instability and chronic low back pain. Now, however, less bone is taken away, with good results and fewer problems. Sometimes ligament or disc material that X-ray studies have shown to be compressing nerves is also removed.

Although decompression surgery does ease pain and improve mobility, it has not proven to be superior to more conservative treatments, such as postural adjustments, losing excess body weight to help reduce stress on spinal structures and the use of anti-inflammatory medicines to decrease swelling and pain around nerves.

Decompression with fusion

Usually done to relieve vertebral slippage (spondylolisthesis; see page 124) associated with spinal stenosis, this procedure combines decompression (see above) with fusion (arthrodesis). This latter involves a bone graft to stabilise the vertebrae, and sometimes the use of metal hardware inserted internally, to provide reinforcement until the bones have knitted together.

Vertebroplasty

Carried out to treat compression fractures of the vertebrae, vertebroplasty helps to strengthen the bones, relieve pain and improve mobility.

Kyphoplasty

A procedure to relieve pain and disability resulting from compression fractures and spinal deformity.

The operation requires the insertion of an inflatable balloon into the body of the vertebra, using X-ray guidance. The balloon is then inflated to help restore some lost height and reverse some of the deformity. Bone cement can then be injected.

Posture Matters

Posture generally refers to the position of your body in space, not only when you sit and stand but also when you walk, kneel or lie down. Posture affects your health and wellbeing because it determines how much stress is placed on body parts such as bones, joints, muscles, ligaments, tendons and spinal discs.

Good posture keeps stress to a minimum and distributes it among various structures according to their ability to bear it. Faulty posture is implicated in every painful condition, including those arising from injury, overuse and degenerative changes.

Body moves

The way in which you move and use your body and its parts in everyday activities is technically referred to as 'body mechanics'. Despite its strength and versatility in health, your body is nevertheless somewhat delicate. If you use it indiscriminately, you may subject it to too much stress, with consequent damage and pain. This is particularly true of the spinal column. Making the right body moves is therefore a prudent preventive measure against back problems.

Sitting

When you sit, you subject your spine to double the stress involved in standing. If you sit a great deal, you therefore put your back at increased risk of backache and associated ailments. To minimise the stress of sitting:

Sit tall, with the crown of your head uppermost, rather than leaning forwards.

Sit on your 'sitting bones' (one under each buttock), rather than on your coccyx (tailbone).

Sit on a chair that gives you good support (if there is no built-in back support, use a prop such as a small cushion or rolled-up towel), with your thighs roughly parallel to the floor, your legs uncrossed and your feet flat on the floor.

Relax your shoulders.

To avert the build up of tension, get up periodically to do gentle body stretches.

On the road

The same rules apply when you're driving a car as when you're sitting at a desk in an office – the way you hold yourself affects the health of your back. Here are tips for motorists to help minimise spinal stress and injury:

Adjust the seat of your vehicle so that you can reach the pedals with your knees slightly bent rather than locked straight.

Sit as far back on your seat as you can to enable you to hold the steering wheel in a secure but relaxed manner. Sit tall but not rigid. Relax your jaw and breathe regularly.

Be sure that your seat provides good neck and back support.

For best protection, use a seat belt with both lap and chest components.

When driving long distances, take periodic breaks: stop at safe rest areas and do gentle tension-relieving exercises.

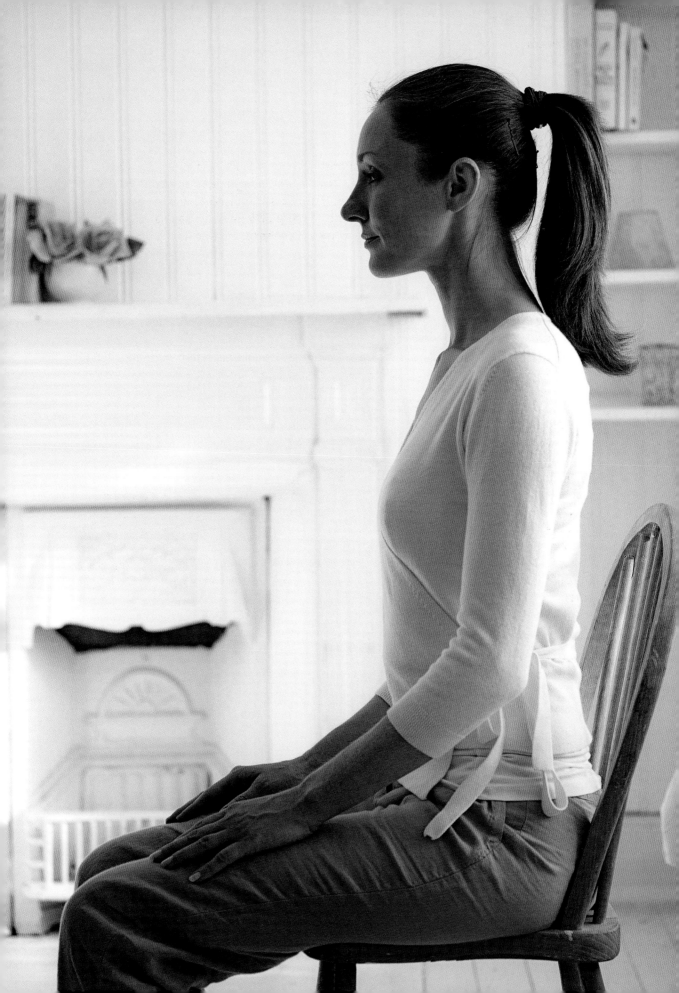

Walking

For strengthening various body structures and for promoting efficient breathing, walking is undoubtedly one of the best exercises. Make it work to your advantage by observing the following:

Begin by standing correctly (see page 55).

Relax your jaw and breathe regularly in synchronisation with an even stride.

Let your arms swing naturally.

Don't jut your chin out; keep your head upright.

Lying down

When you lie down, you give your spine relief from day-to-day stresses, including pressure on intervertebral discs.

It is best to lie on your side or on your back (supine). If you do have to lie on your abdomen (prone), insert a flat pillow or cushion under your abdomen and possibly one under your feet also. The former helps to prevent an exaggerated spinal arch at the small of your back (lordosis).

When you lie on your back, place a pillow or cushion under your knees to avoid possible back strain. Use only one pillow on which to rest your head, unless this is not comfortable for you. If you're just having a quick rest, try rolling a towel like a sausage and placing it under your neck for support and stability.

In a supine position, try leaning one knee against the other and resting separated feet flat on the surface on which you are lying.

For short periods of relaxation, lie on a carpeted floor and rest your feet on a padded chair seat. Your knee and hip joints should each form about a 90-degree angle. Rest your head on a pillow or cushion.

Periodically lie on your side with your hip and knee joints bent. Place one pillow under your head and one each between your knees and ankles. This position relaxes the back, and the pillows or cushions ease the pressure of one bony prominence on the other.

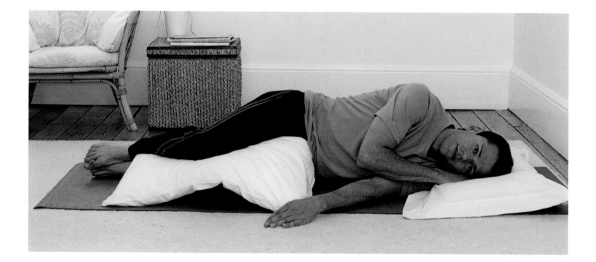

Getting up safely

When preparing to get up from lying supine,
avoid coming straight forwards. Instead:

Roll onto your side; bend your knees and bring
them closer to your body.

Push yourself onto your hip.

Carefully pivot yourself until you are sitting
securely on your bottom.

Take a few slow, smooth breaths and slowly
stand up.

Synchronise all your movements with regular,
attentive breathing.

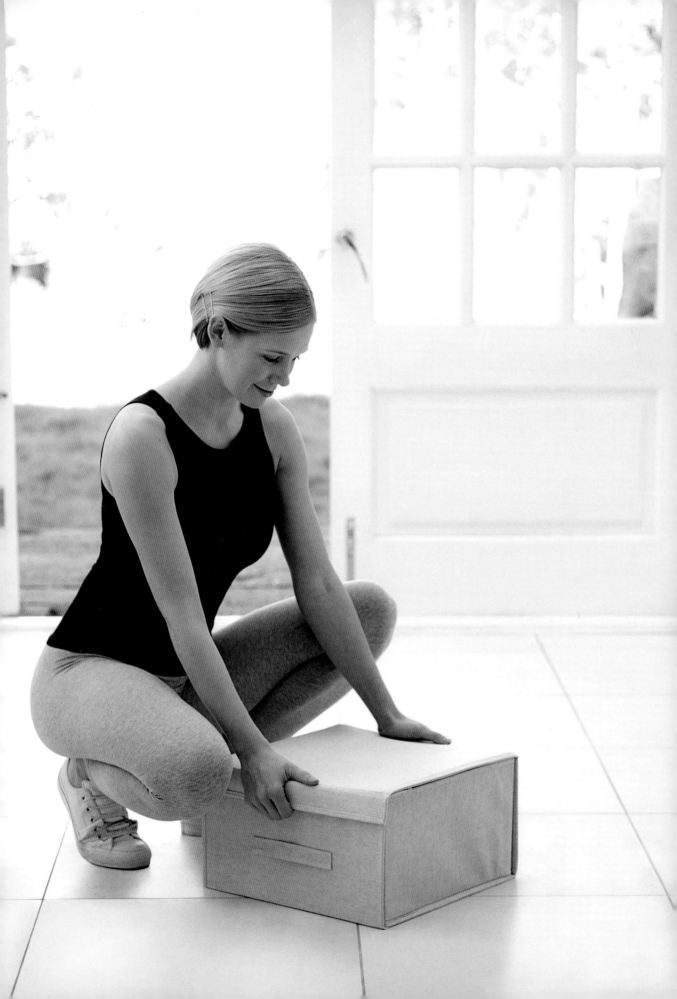

Bending and lifting

Here are six simple rules to help prevent back injury when you bend and lift even moderately heavy objects:

Stand close to the object to be lifted, with your feet comfortably apart for good balance.

Keep your head and torso erect.

Put one foot slightly behind the other and bend your knees to lower your body; maintain good posture.

With arms slightly bent at the elbows and wrists kept straight, securely hold the object to be lifted; keep it close to the centre of your body.

Keep your abdomen and chin tucked in, and use your legs rather than your back to do the lifting.

Bend your knees and lift with ease, in synchronisation with regular breathing – execute a gradual, smooth lift and avoid jerking.

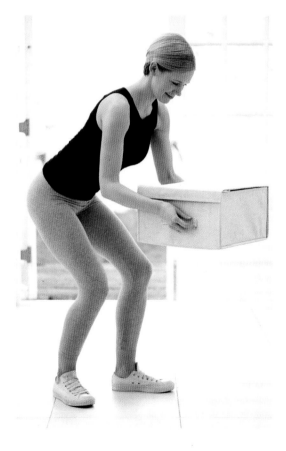 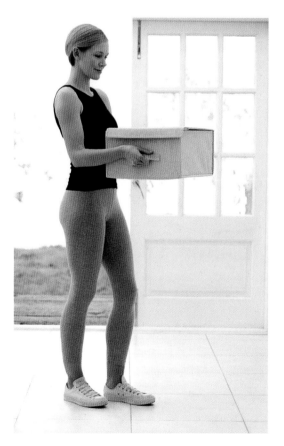

Housework

To decrease your risk of back ailments, consider applying the 'divide and conquer' principle when doing household chores.

Do only a few each day rather than try to accomplish them all at once.

Take frequent breaks to practise tension-relieving exercises (see pages 62–70).

Ask family members to help with some of the more demanding jobs.

Always pay careful attention to your posture and body mechanics, no matter what a task entails.

Avoid sudden twisting motions, as may occur when you transfer laundry from washer to dryer, for example. Instead of twisting your upper body, move your feet and swivel your whole body.

Avoid doing two actions at once, such as lifting and twisting.

Don't stand in a fixed position for a long time. It is stressful for the neck and back muscles. Rest your foot on a prop if you can, such as a box or footstool, and periodically shift your weight from side to side.

When working at a counter, table, ironing board or similar flat surface, be sure that its height allows you to work without strain. Ideally, the surface should be near your hip, and you should be able to work with your elbows comfortably bent. Alternatively, you can sit on a high stool to take the weight off your feet and so reduce back fatigue.

During seated activities such as eating or writing, avoid leaning forwards. This stresses the neck, back and shoulders. Instead, place your chair comfortably close to the table.

To clean a bathtub, attend to a small child or do something else that requires you to lower your body, kneel down or squat rather than bending forwards from a standing position.

Instead of carrying one heavy load of laundry up or down the stairs, divide it into two or more parts and make a separate trip for eac

To vacuum-clean a carpet or mop a floor, try using a lunging technique: keep your torso erect and use your legs and arms to do most of the work. If possible, use a long-handled vacuum cleaner.

To tuck bed sheets under a mattress, kneel down, rather than bend over. For far corners, rest one knee on the bed and brace yourself with one hand to take pressure off your back. If at all possible, position the bed so that you have easy access to all sides of it, and use fitted sheets and a duvet to keep bed-making and back strain to a minimum.

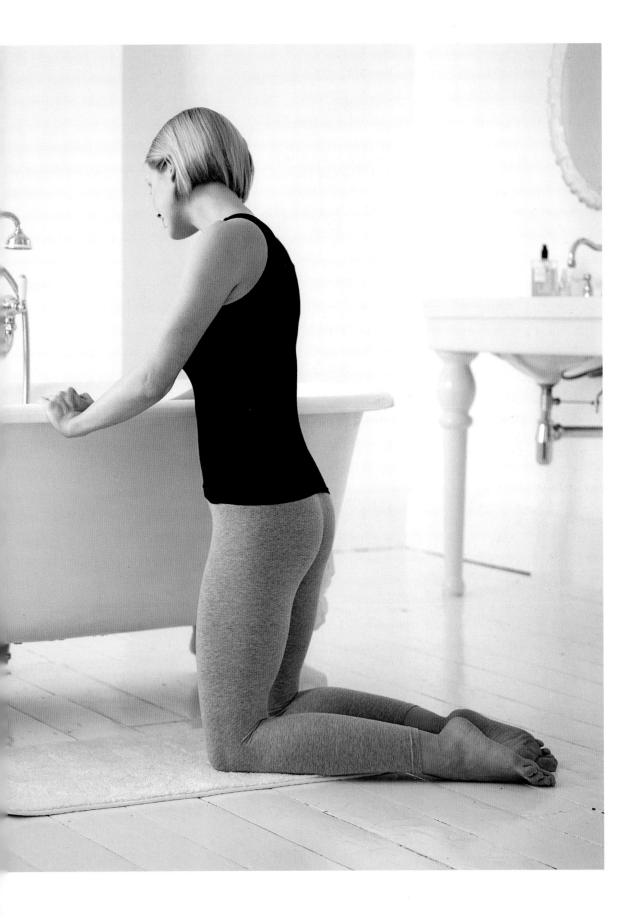

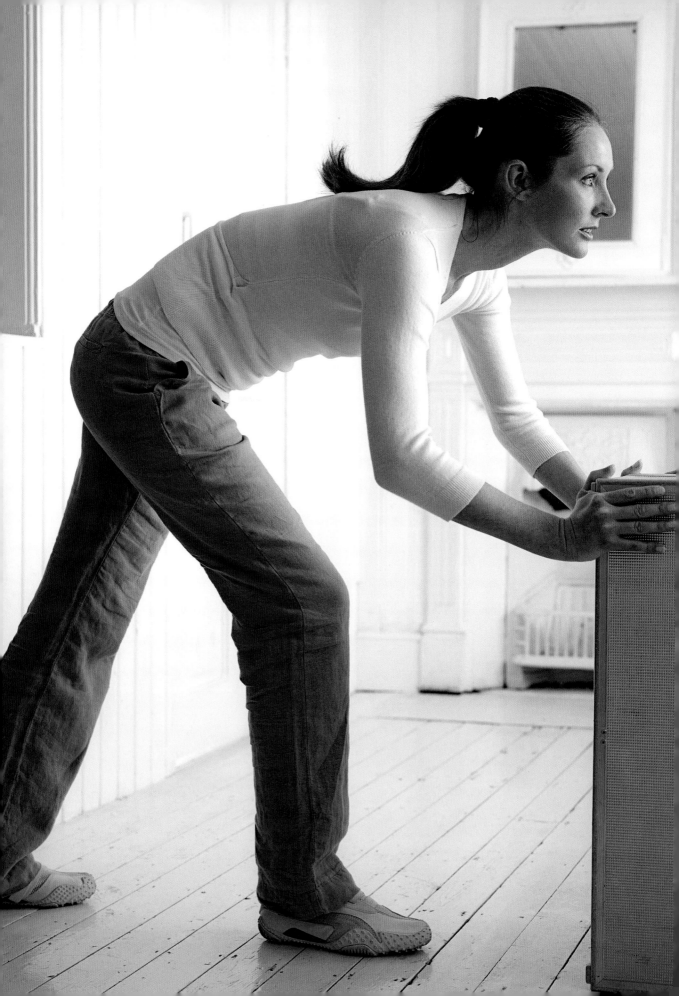

In the workplace

Prolonged sitting at a desk or computer can take a toll on your back. If the design and arrangement of the furniture are incompatible with good posture and body mechanics, the risk of back problems increases. You can do your part, however, to minimise stress on spinal structures and so help to prevent back-related difficulties.

Organise your work station so that you can easily reach frequently used items with a minimum of bending, twisting and reaching.

The height of your chair seat should allow you to rest your feet flat on the floor, with your lower legs roughly vertical, and the length of your thighs well supported.

Ideally, your chair should have built-in support for your shoulders and lower back.

Avoid crossing your legs, since this tilts your pelvis forwards, increases the normal lumbar curve of the spine and strains the back.

To avoid your having to look downwards, the centre of your computer should be about level with your eyes. This helps to prevent strain on the neck and upper back muscles.

Your keyboard should be located at a height to allow your upper arms to be relaxed at your sides and your forearms, wrists and hands to be in a straight line.

Do not wedge the telephone handset between your ear and shoulder to free your hands. It strains the neck muscles. Use a headset or speaker phone instead.

To prevent cumulative stress disorders (repetitive strain injury), get up periodically and do simple tension-relieving exercises, such as the Neck Stretches and Shoulder Rolls on pages 62–65.

Pushing and pulling

Push instead of pull whenever you can when moving heavy objects such as items of furniture and loaded wheelbarrows. To minimise stress:

Keep your knees slightly bent rather than rigid.

Keep your head, neck and back in good alignment.

Working in the garden

Before attempting to do any vigorous outdoor work shortly after getting out of bed in the morning, be sure to warm up your body properly (see page 62). During sleep, the centre of your spinal discs (page 12) absorb extra fluid and swell somewhat. This is normally counteracted by the pressing of vertebrae on discs during regular activities. Immediately following a night in bed, however, the swollen discs are more vulnerable to damage than they are later in the day. (This caution also applies to strenuous indoor work.)

Squat or kneel down to do as many chores as you can, such as transplanting seedlings or pulling up weeds, rather than bending forwards at the waist.

Vary your tasks, rather than spending long periods on one at a time. For example, alternate digging with pruning or raking leaves.

To avoid straining your neck and back, be very careful not to overreach – for example, when pruning high branches.

Put into practise the general rules of correct bending and lifting (page 47).

To avoid the buildup of muscle tension and fatigue, take short periodic breaks to do simple stretching exercises.

Hygiene and grooming

Particularly when you're in a hurry to get to work or keep an appointment, you may be less than careful and so risk subjecting your neck or back to injury. To lessen the chances of mishap, be aware of the following points when attending to your personal hygiene and grooming.

Avoid washing your hair in a sink or while bending over a bathtub.

To dry your feet, sit on a stool or other prop and bring one foot at a time towards you.

Stand tall or sit down to shave or apply make-up. Position the mirror so that either can be done with complete ease.

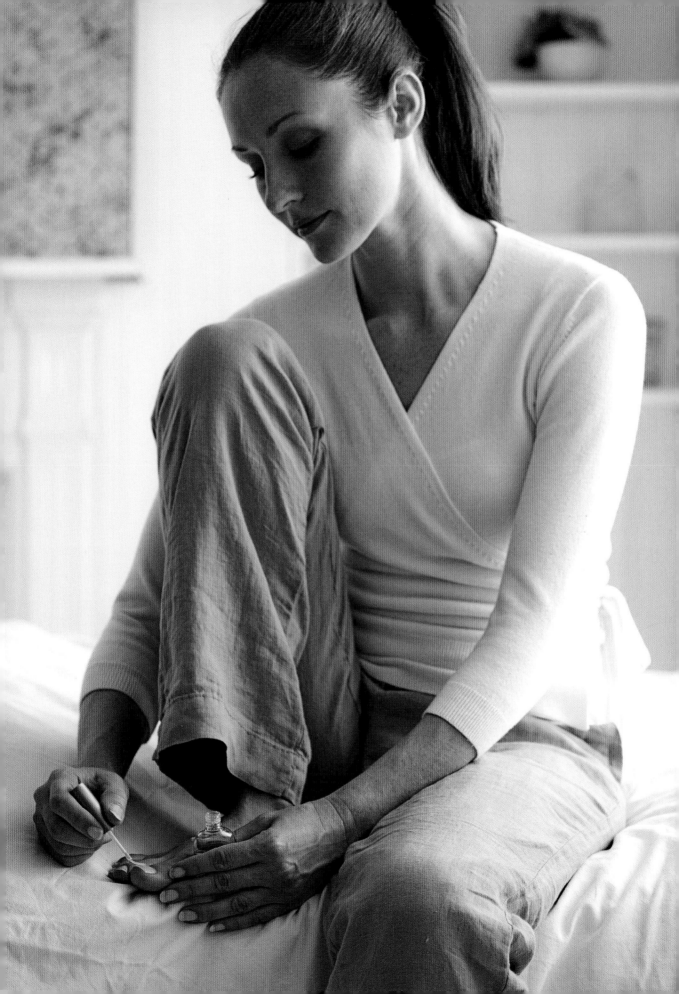

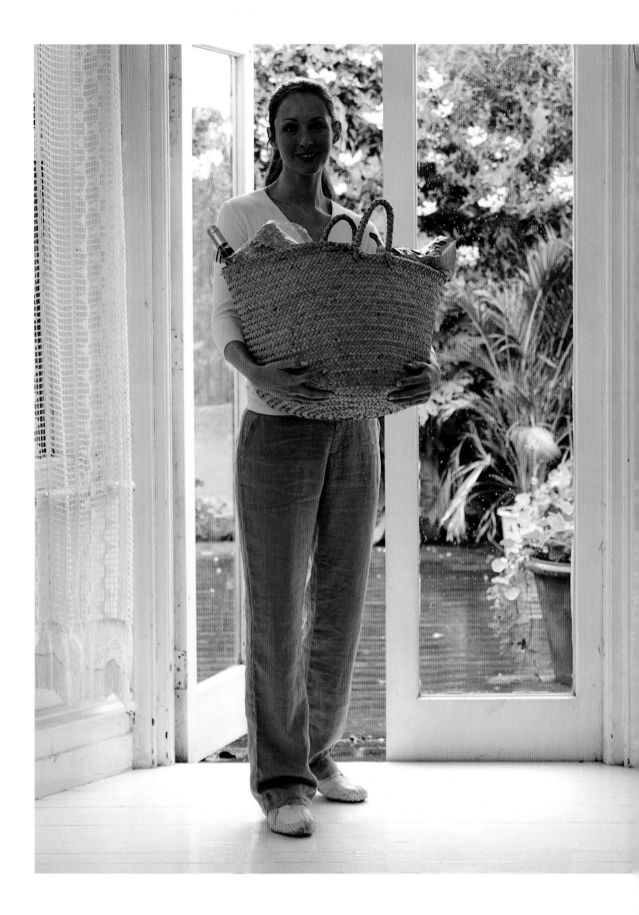

Carrying

Carrying objects incorrectly is one way of disrupting the body's symmetry and balance. It subjects the spine and its associated structures to unnecessary stress. To prevent or minimise this risk:

Divide heavy loads into two or more lighter ones, even if you have to make an extra trip.

Hold the objects close to your body.

Ask someone to help you, or use a cart or trolley.

Avoid carrying a heavy object, such as a large bag, on only one side of your body. Instead, divide the contents into two parts, if you can, and carry one in each hand or arm.

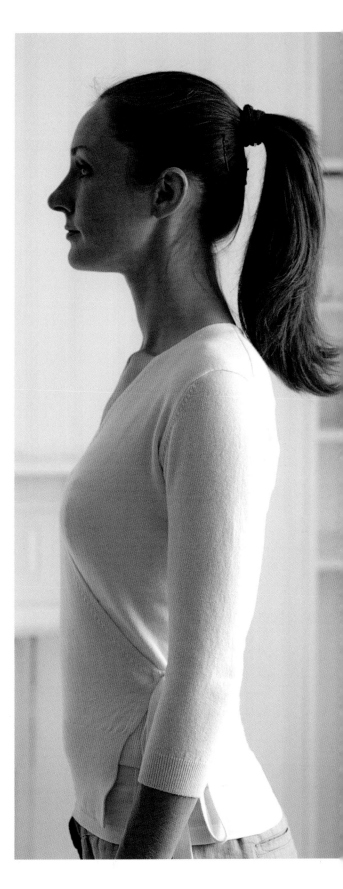

Standing

Even when you stand correctly, tremendous pressure is placed on your lumbar discs. When standing for any length of time is unavoidable, however, rest one foot on a prop. In addition:

Stand tall, with the crown of your head uppermost, your shoulders relaxed and your body weight equally distributed between your feet.

Don't lock your knee joints; keep them somewhat relaxed.

Sport

Having a back ailment does not necessarily mean that you shouldn't participate in sport. You should, however, be sure to warm up properly before your chosen activity and cool down sufficiently afterwards. In addition, try to stay conditioned at all times. Sports injuries tend to occur not because of the sport itself, but rather because of poor technique and inadequate conditioning and warming up.

Swimming

In general, this is one of the best exercises for people with certain back problems. The side stroke is usually the best choice, provided you learn to alternate sides. The crawl, butterfly and breast strokes are not advised, however, since they require arching the back, which could aggravate existing difficulties. The back stroke may be tried, provided there is no overarching of the lower back. Before you swim, be sure to do some stretching and strengthening exercises.

Racquet sports

Tennis and other racquet sports require flexible leg and hip joints. They also involve twisting movements that tax spinal and sacroiliac joints. Combined with vigorous swings and asymmetrical upper body action, all these moves can put the spine and associated structures at risk of injury.

Be sure to maintain flexibility, particularly of the upper body, and to do stretching exercises before and after each game. If you are a beginner, you might also consider taking a few lessons from a professional to learn good technique. Remember, too, to squat when picking up the ball, rather than bending forwards.

Jogging

Do wear proper shoes and avoid jogging on hard surfaces, which can transmit vibration to the spine and cause damage to discs and other spinal components. Being overweight increases this risk, so it would be prudent to keep this in check. Remember to do warm ups before you run, maintain good posture and cool down properly.

Downhill skiing

Maintaining bodily strength and flexibility is crucial to safe, enjoyable downhill skiing. Tightness of the leg, hip, shoulder and spinal joints could set the scene for back injury. Warm up and cool down exercises are also imperative.

Golf

Like racquet and other sports that involve asymmetric body moves and twisting, golf can place heavy demands on the spine and related structures. To minimise stress:

Do maintain bodily strength and flexibility through regular appropriate exercise.

Warm up adequately before the game and cool down properly afterwards.

Wear well-fitting and supportive shoes.

If you're a beginner, consider taking lessons from a professional, to learn correct technique.

In general

The key to good posture is overall fitness. But no single exercise programme will give you good posture if you do not habitually practise good habits in the way you hold yourself and carry out daily activities. Habitually holding yourself elegantly but not stiffly, and moving your body and its parts in accord with their structure and functions will minimise the stress to which they are subjected. This will, in the long term, do more to help prevent back ailments than any other single measure you can take. And the effort will be well worth your while.

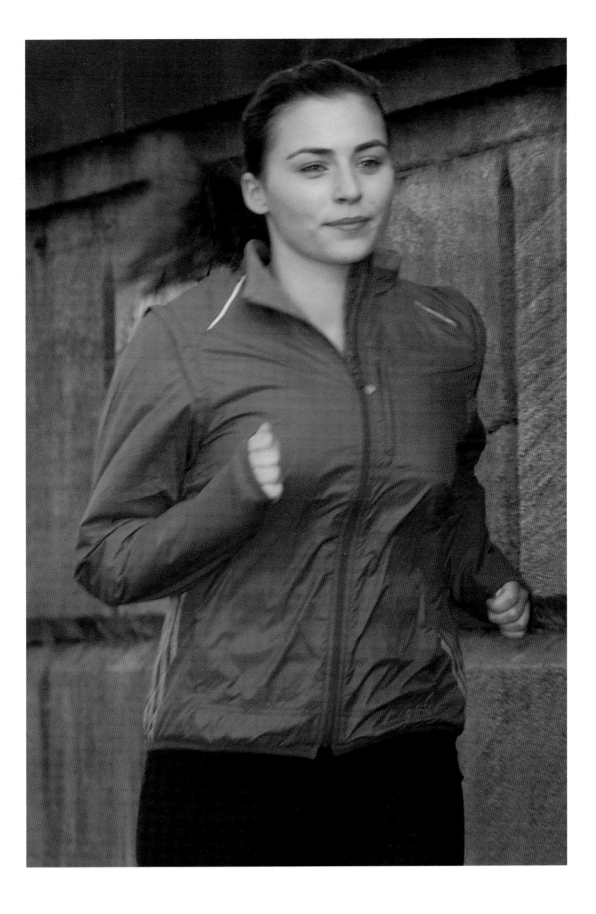

Healing Back Exercises

One of the most powerful adjuncts to any treatment for relieving pain is, without a doubt, regular exercise. The weakness that often accompanies musculoskeletal pain can, in part, be altered by exercise.

Why exercise?

Exercise has many benefits, not only for maintaining a healthy body, but also for helping the body cope with pain. Exercise can help to heal back ailments and prevent their occurrence and can significantly reduce stress.

The benefits

Increases the level of endorphins, the body's own morphine-like pain relievers, the action of which is not unlike that of acupuncture and electrical nerve stimulation, or TENS.

Increases the production of synovial fluid in joints (such as the facet joints), which helps to reduce wear and tear.

Increases the tensile strength of tendons and ligaments, making them better able to resist strain and tissue damage.

Strengthens joints and muscles, rendering them less vulnerable to injury.

Decreases the risk of osteoporosis, which makes bones more susceptible to fracture.

Improves coordination and balance, which help to protect against falls and consequent injury.

Is one of the best tools for coping with stress.

Preparing for exercise

Before you attempt to do the exercises in this book, or to embark on any exercise programme, please first check with your doctor or other professional health-care provider. This precaution is especially important if you are recovering from an injury or from surgery, if you have osteoporosis or other health disorder, if you are pregnant, or if you have not engaged in regular exercise for some time.

When, where and how

For best results, try to do some exercise every day. There are many simple stretches you can integrate into everyday activities no matter how busy you are (see opposite). If this is not possible, try to do some exercise at least every other day – practising regularly is important for maintaining the good results gained from the previous session.

Try not to exercise too close to meal times as it may interfere with digestion.

Make sure that your exercise area is free of obstruction and practise whenever possible on a non-skid surface.

Remove any personal items that can cause injury.

Wear clothing that allows you to move and breathe easily. If you wear shoes, they should provide good traction.

Practise slowly and attentively, in synchronisation with regular breathing.

Cautions

At the first hint of pain while exercising, stop. You may be performing the movement incorrectly, or the exercise may not be appropriate for you at this time.

If you have osteoporosis, some forward-bending exercises are best avoided because of possible compression fracture of spinal bones. Check with your doctor.

Pregnant women with a history of miscarriage should avoid the exercises in this book during the first trimester (three months). Check with your doctor. During pregnancy, omit exercises done in the prone position (lying on the abdomen). After the first trimester, avoid exercises requiring you to lie flat on your back: this position can restrict the delivery of blood and oxygen to mother and foetus by placing pressure on the mother's vena cava (principal vein) draining the lower body.

Stretching

Chief among the benefits to be derived from daily stretching are injury prevention and faster recovery from exercise. A regular programme of stretching exercises will increase the range of motion of your spinal and other joints. It will also facilitate the delivery of nutrients to and removal of wastes from the body's tissues and promote healing.

When and how

Try to do some stretches every day and repeat each about three times.

Make sure your stretches are slow and smooth and synchronised with regular breathing.

Hold (maintain) each stretch for 5 to 20 seconds, but no longer than 90 seconds.

Warm ups

Regardless of how short your exercise programme is, a brief warm up period is imperative. Warm ups slightly increase body temperature, reduce stiffness and improve circulation. They help to prevent muscular pulls and strains when you do the main exercises or engage in sports or other strenuous activities.

When and how

Spend at least five minutes warming up; longer for more vigorous endeavours.

Do your warm ups slowly and attentively, maintain good posture and breathe regularly.

Some of the warm ups in this chapter can be integrated into daily activities to prevent or reduce tension build-up. You can, for example, do Shoulder Rolls (below) or Neck Stretches (page 64) during short breaks from prolonged sitting at a desk or computer.

Whenever the word 'mat' is used in the instructions, it refers to the surface on which you are doing the exercise.

The word 'hold' means 'maintain' a stretch or completed exercise. The length of time for holding the position will vary with your level of functioning. The number of times to repeat an exercise will also depend on your general condition. Keep these to a minimum if you have not exercised for some time or if you are recovering from an illness or from surgery. Check with your doctor or physiotherapist.

Shoulder Rolls

What they do	How to do them
Enhance the effects of the Neck Stretches	1 Sit or stand tall. Relax your hands. Relax your jaw and breathe regularly.
Condition the muscles of the upper back	2 Slowly and smoothly rotate your shoulders in a backward to forwards motion three or more times.
Keep the shoulder joints freely moving	3 Repeat the Shoulder Rolls three or more times in the opposite direction. Rest.
Prevent tension build-up in the upper back	

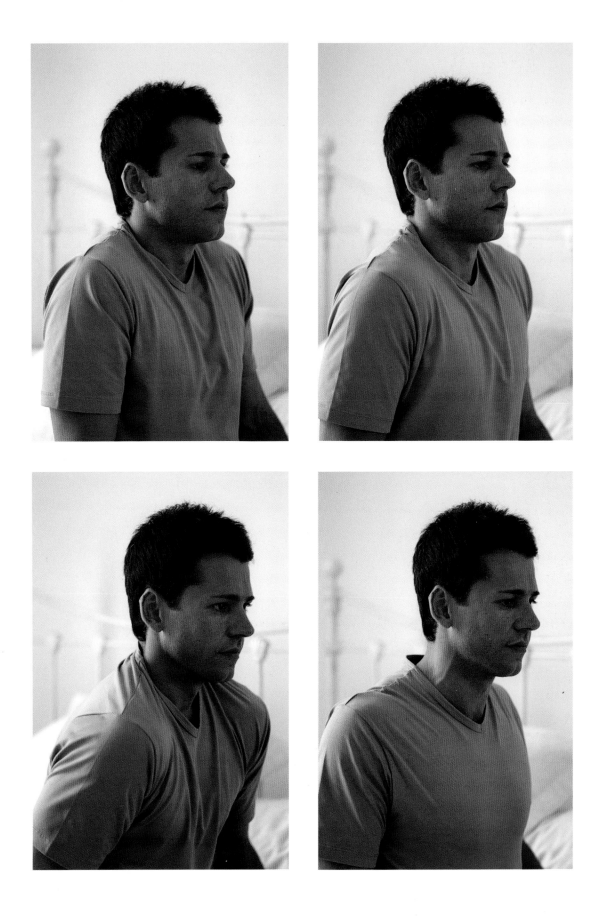

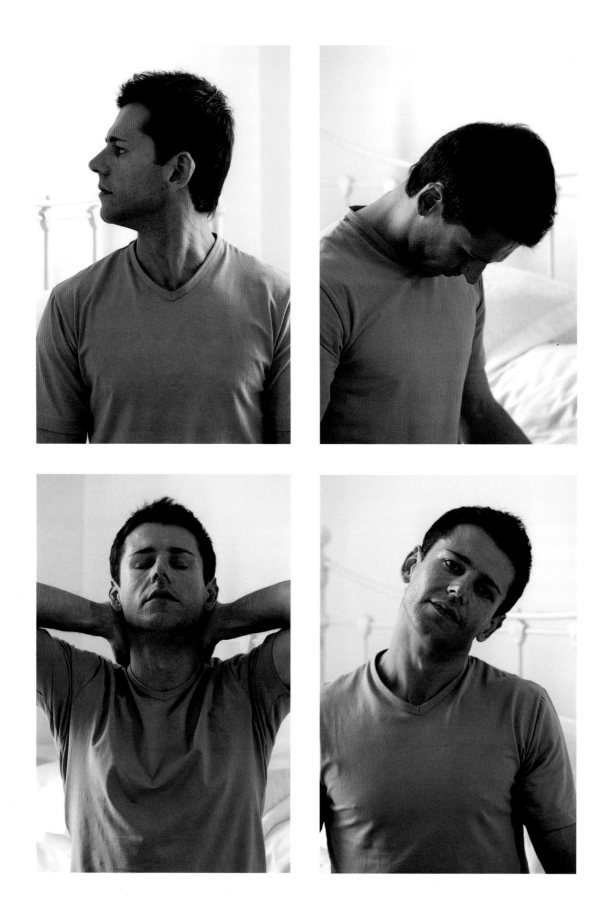

Neck Stretches

What they do

Keep the cervical (neck) part of the spine flexible and counteract stiffness

Contribute to a healthy spinal circulation

Prevent tension build-up in the neck

Strengthen neck muscles

How to do them

1 Sit or stand tall. Relax your shoulders and hands. Relax your jaw and breathe regularly.

2 Slowly and smoothly turn your head as far to the left as you comfortably can. Hold the neck stretch for five or more seconds.

3 Turn your head slowly and smoothly to the right as far as you comfortably can. Hold the neck stretch for five or more seconds.

4 Repeat these two moves (steps 2 and 3) two or more times.

5 Gently supporting the back of your neck with your hands, slowly and carefully tilt your head backwards. Hold the neck stretch for five or more seconds.

6 Relax your hands and slowly and carefully tilt your chin towards your chest. Hold the neck stretch for five or more seconds.

7 Repeat these two moves (steps 5 and 6) two or more times before returning to your starting position.

8 Slowly and smoothly tilt your left ear towards your left shoulder to stretch the right side of your neck. Hold the stretch for five or more seconds.

9 Repeat the sideways neck stretch (step 8) on the other side.

10 Repeat these two neck stretches (steps 8 and 9) two or more times before resuming your starting position, with head upright and facing forwards. Rest.

The next set of warm ups are for the lumbar part of the spine, at the small of the back.

Pelvic Tilt

What it does

Strengthens the lower back

Strengthens the abdominal muscles

Keeps the spine flexible

Relieves spinal stiffness and minor backaches

How to do it

1 Sit on a chair or stand with your back to a wall or other prop. Maintain good posture, relax your jaw and breathe regularly.

2 On an exhalation, press the back of your waist towards or against the back of the chair or other prop. Hold the pressure as long as your exhalation lasts. This will gently tilt your pelvis.

3 Inhale and relax, then repeat the exercise (steps 2 and 3) two or more times. Rest.

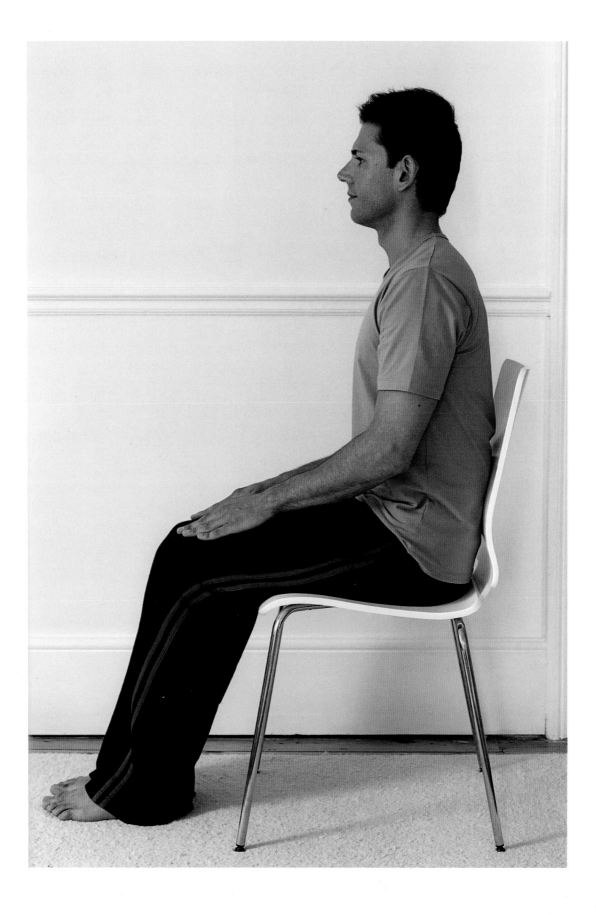

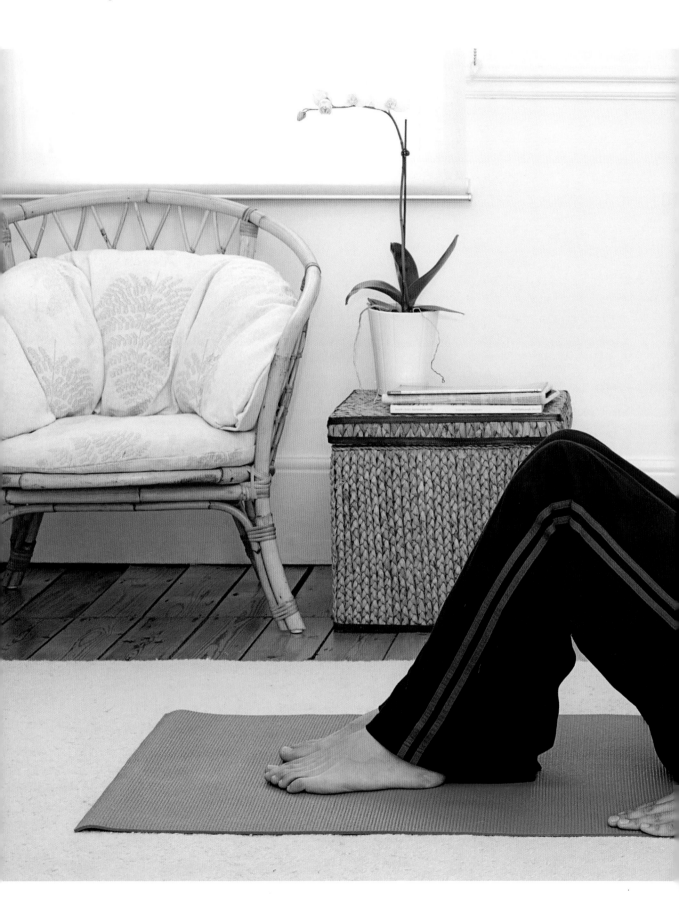

Variation
Pelvic Tilt

What it does

Strengthens the lower back

Strengthens the abdominal muscles

Keeps the spine flexible

Relieves spinal stiffness and minor backaches

How to do it

1 Lie on your back, bend your knees and rest your feet flat on the mat. Relax your arms at your sides.

2 On an exhalation, press the small of your back towards or against the mat. Hold the downward pressure as long as your exhalation lasts.

3 Inhale and relax your back, then repeat the exercise (steps 2 and 3) two or more times. Rest.

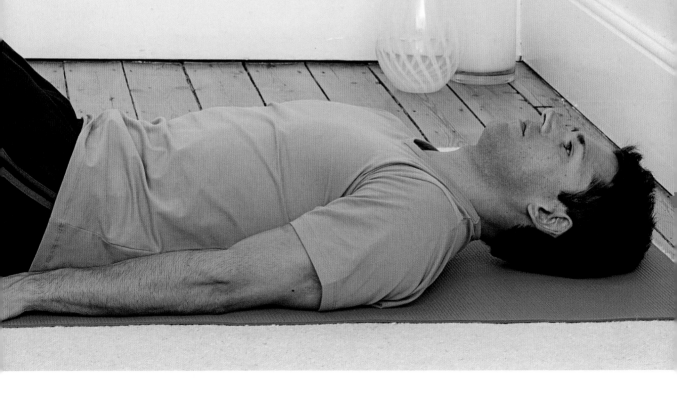

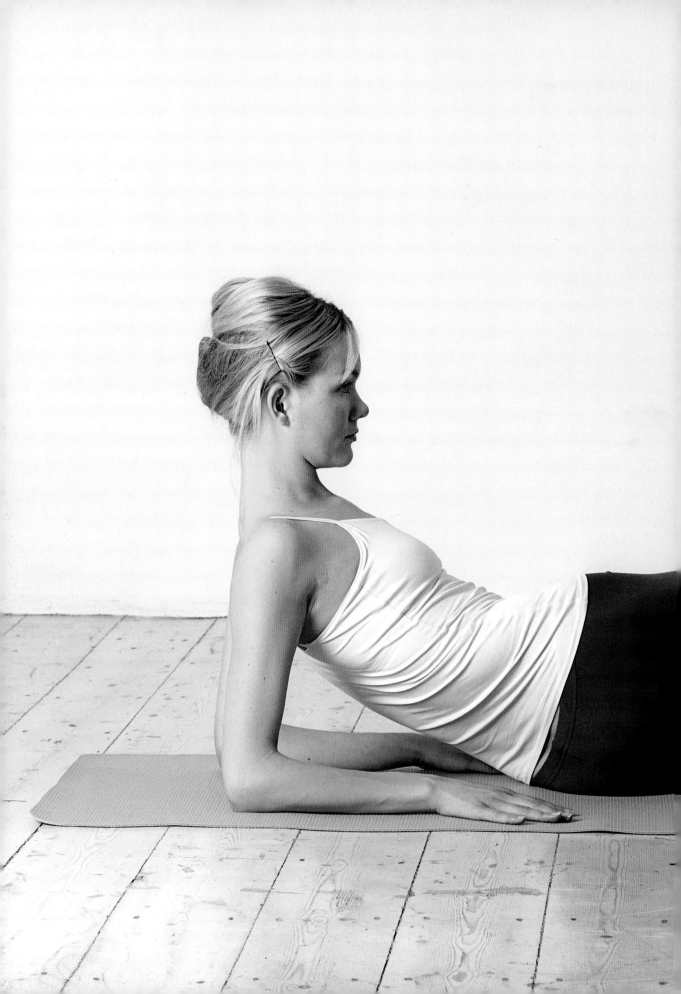

Reclining Twist

What it does

Helps to keep the lower spine flexible

Conditions the lower back muscles

Firms and strengthens the oblique and transverse abdominal muscles (page 13)

How to do it

1 Sit on your mat. Bend your knees and rest the soles of your feet on the mat. Lean backwards and prop yourself up on your elbows. Relax your jaw and breathe regularly.

2 Bring your knees towards your body. Alternately tilt your knees, as a unit, to left and right in synchronisation with regular breathing.

3 Repeat these movements (step 2) five or more times on each side before resuming your starting position. Rest.

CAUTION

Pregnant women and individuals with osteoporosis should omit this exercise.

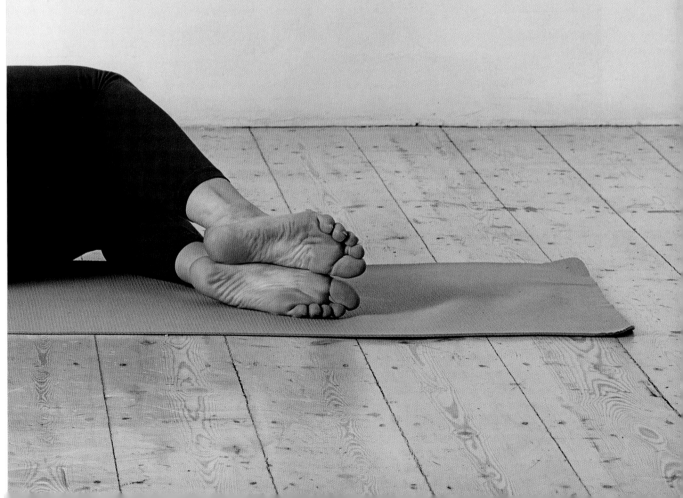

Healing back sequence

Here is a sequence of exercises that is manageable for most people. It is designed to make the transition from one exercise to the other smooth and logical. As described, it takes about ten minutes to do altogether, including the warm ups on pages 62–73, depending on the number of repetitions and on how long you hold each finished position or final stretch. Try to do the exercises in the order given. If this is not quite right for you, modify the sequence for maximum comfort. You can also practise any of the exercises individually whenever it suits you. Do each one slowly, smoothly and attentively, and synchronise your movements with regular breathing, with jaw relaxed.

Getting up safely from lying supine

When doing these exercises, and indeed at any other time, to avoid injuring your back, never get up from a supine (lying on the back) position by bolting straight forwards. Instead, follow these simple steps:

Check that you are breathing regularly. Synchronise your breathing with every
   move you make.
Roll onto your side, bend your knees and bring them closer to your torso.
Use your hands to help push you onto your hip.
Carefully manoeuvre yourself until you are sitting evenly on your bottom.
Sit quietly for a few seconds before standing up or assuming another position.

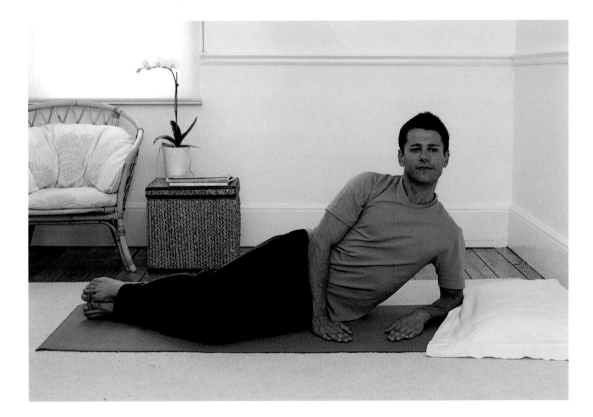

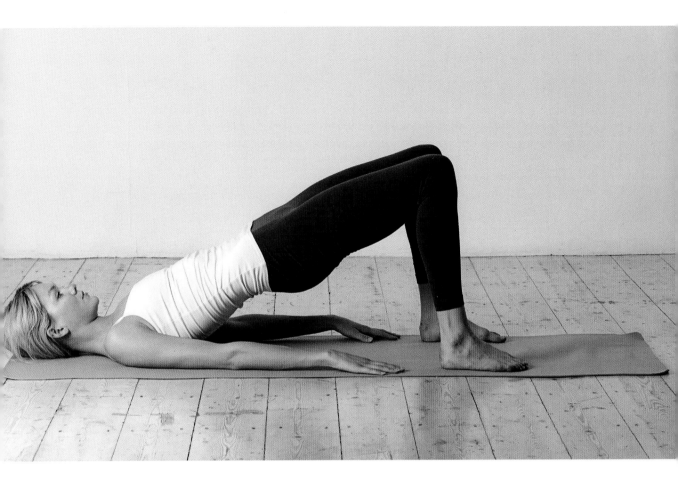

The Bridge

What it does

Tones the muscles at the front and back of the body

Helps to keep the spine flexible

How to do it

1 Lie on your back on a mat. Bend your knees and rest your feet flat and comfortably close to your body. Breathe regularly. Relax your arms at your sides.

2 On an inhalation slowly raise your torso, from hips to upper back.

3 When you have reached your comfortable limit, hold the posture for five or more seconds while breathing regularly.

4 To return to your starting position, slowly and smoothly lower your torso from top to bottom. Stretch out your legs and rest.

5 You may repeat the exercise once or twice.

Alternate Leg Raise

What it does

Strengthens the back muscles

Strengthens the abdominal muscles

Gently stretches the hamstring muscles, which are secondary back supports (page 13)

How to do it

1 Lie on your back on a mat, with legs stretched out in front. Relax your arms at your sides. Breathe regularly.

2 Bend one leg and rest the sole of the foot on the mat.

3 Raise the other leg slowly and with control, a few inches/centimetres from the mat. You may flex your ankle to point your toes upwards.

4 Hold the raised-leg posture for five or more seconds while breathing regularly.

5 Lower and relax the leg.

6 Repeat steps 3 to 5 two or more times.

7 Repeat the exercise (steps 3 to 5) three or more times with the other leg. Rest.

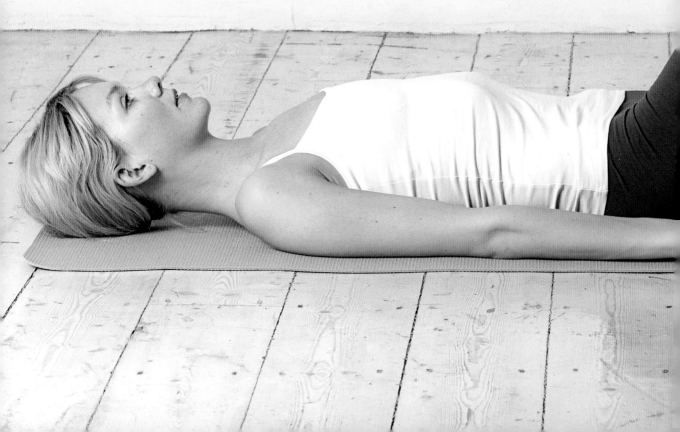

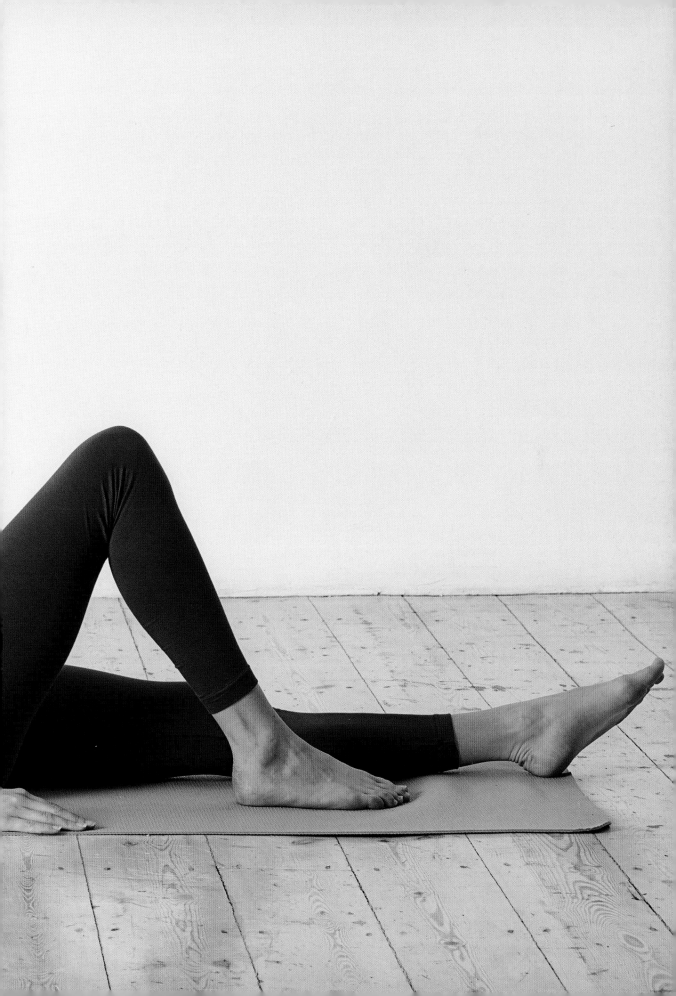

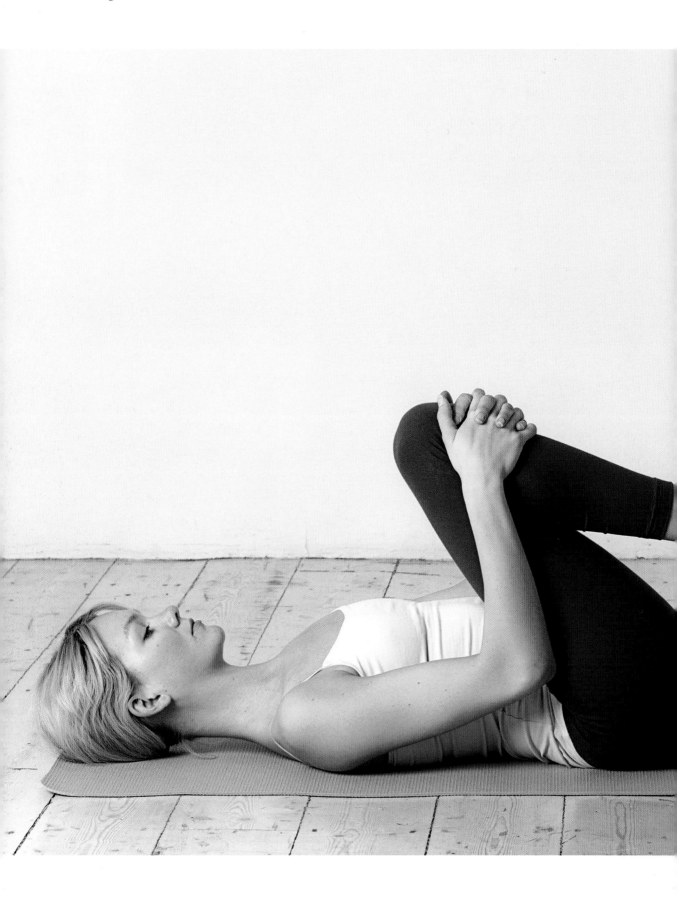

Alternate
Knee Hug

What it does

Tones the back and abdominal muscles

Relaxes the back and relieves minor backaches

Helps to keep the spine flexible

How to do it

1   Lie on your back on a mat, with your legs stretched out in front. Breathe regularly.

2   Bend one leg and bring the knee towards you. Hold it in place with your hands for five or more seconds while breathing regularly.

3   Relax your hands and stretch out your leg.

4   Repeat steps 2 and 3 two or more times.

5   Repeat the exercise (steps 2 and 3) three or more times with the other leg. Rest.

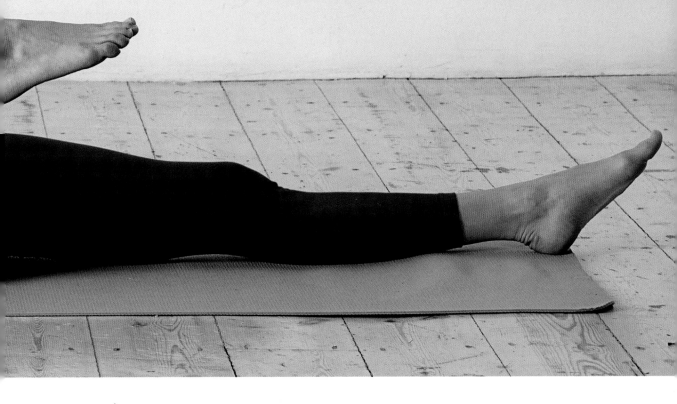

Curl Up

What it does

Tones and strengthens abdominal muscles and so indirectly gives support to back muscles

Helps to keep the spine flexible

A safer alternative to some conventional sit-ups

How to do it

1 Lie on your back on a mat, with your legs stretched out in front. Breathe regularly.

2 Bend your knees until you can rest the soles of your feet flat on the mat.

3 Rest your palms on your thighs.

4 Carefully lift up your head and as much of your upper back as you comfortably can. As you do so, your hands will slide towards your knees. Keep your gaze on your hands.

5 Hold the curl-up for five seconds or more while breathing regularly.

6 Curl back onto the mat and stretch out your legs to resume your starting position. Relax your arms at your sides. Rest.

7 You may repeat the exercise (steps 2 to 6) once or twice.

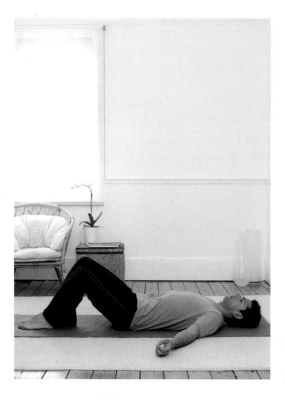 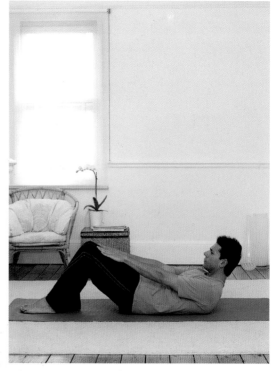

Diagonal
Curl Up

What it does

Complements the Curl Up
(opposite)

Tones and strengthens
abdominal muscles and so
reinforces back muscles

Helps to keep the spine flexible

How to do it

1 Lie on your back on a mat, with your legs stretched out in front.
Breathe regularly.

2 Bend your knees until you can rest the soles of your feet flat on
the mat.

3 Carefully lift up your head to begin a curl-up but, instead of
continuing forwards, reach with both arms to the outside of
your bent legs to execute a diagonal curl-up.

4 Hold the posture for five seconds or more while breathing
regularly. Curl back onto the mat and stretch out your legs to
resume your starting position. Relax your arms at your sides.
Rest.

5 Repeat the exercise on the opposite side (steps 2 to 5). Rest.

6 You may repeat the entire sequence (steps 2 to 6) once or twice.

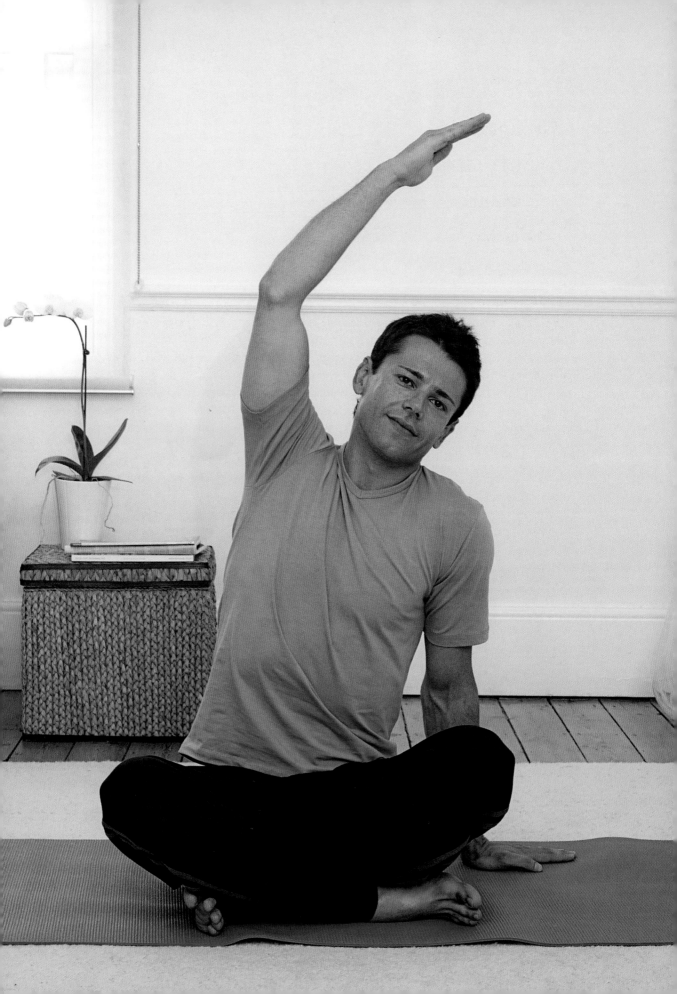

Sideways Stretch

What it does

Tones back and abdominal muscles

Complements the Curl-Up exercises (pages 80–81)

Complements the Spinal Twist (page 84)

Facilitates free movement of the ribcage for more efficient breathing (see ankylosing spondylitis on page 122)

How to do it

1 Sit tall and fold your legs inwards. Breathe regularly.

2 Rest the palm of your right hand on the mat beside your hip.

3 Stretch your left arm straight upwards.

4 Keeping your lower body still, bend and stretch your upper torso towards the right as far as you comfortably can while exhaling.

5 Hold the stretch for five or more seconds while breathing regularly.

6 Inhale and return to your starting position. Rest briefly.

7 Repeat the exercise (steps 2 to 6) on the other side (substitute the word 'left' for 'right' and vice versa).

8 Repeat the entire exercise (steps 2 to 7) two or more times. Rest.

Spinal Twist Variation

What it does

Allows maximum torsion (twisting) of the spine to both sides and so provides a gentle, therapeutic massage to nerves branching from the spinal column

Helps to keep the spine flexible

Tones the lower back muscles

Tones the transverse and oblique abdominal muscles (page 13)

Enhances spinal circulation

How to do it

1 Sit tall on your heels, Japanese style. Breathe regularly.

2 Slowly rotate your upper body to the right as you exhale.

3 Hold on to the outside of your right thigh with your left hand. Rest your right hand on your lower back. Look over your right shoulder.

4 Hold the posture for five or more seconds while breathing regularly.

5 Slowly resume your starting position. Rest briefly.

6 Repeat the exercise (steps 2 to 5) on the other side (substitute the word 'left' for 'right' and vice versa).

7 Repeat the entire exercise (steps 2 to 6) once or twice. Rest.

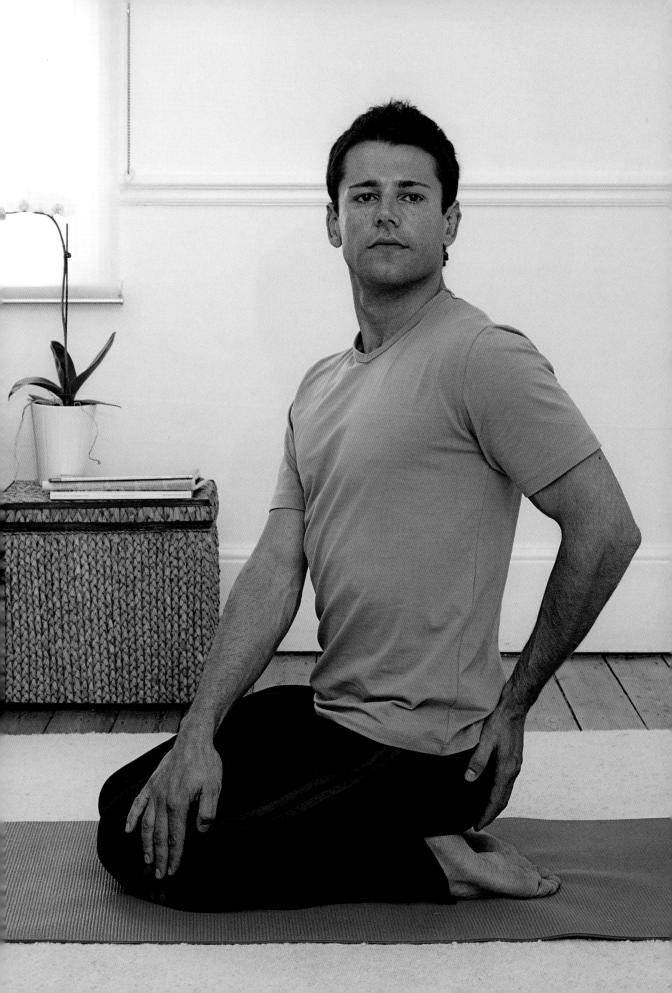

Squatting Posture

What it does

Eases pressure on spinal discs through gentle traction

Improves spinal flexibility

Tones back and abdominal muscles

How to do it

1 From a standing position, lower your body as if to sit on your heels. Try to keep your feet flat on the mat. Breathe regularly.

2 Hold the posture for five seconds or more.

3 Stand up again.

4 Repeat the exercise (steps 2 and 3) two or more times. Rest.

NOTE

Incorporate squatting into daily activities (see pages 42–55).

Dog Stretch

What it does

Gives a therapeutic stretch to the back and the legs, which are secondary back supports

Relieves fatigue in the back and legs

Helps to maintain the elasticity of the hamstrings: when these muscles shorten, they affect the angle of pelvic tilt and so influence posture

How to do it

1 Start in an all-fours position, on hands and knees, with arms sloping slightly forwards. Breathe regularly.

2 Rock forwards somewhat, raise your knees and straighten your legs. Aim your heels towards the mat but do not strain. Straighten your arms and keep your head down.

3 Hold the posture for five or more seconds while breathing regularly.

4 Rock forwards gently and ease into your starting position.

5 Sit on your heels and rest.

6 You may repeat the exercise (steps 1 to 5) once or twice.

CAUTION

Do not practise this posture if you have high blood pressure, or a heart condition or other disorder that produces feelings of lightheadedness or dizziness when you hang your head down. Instead, try the alternative exercise that follows.

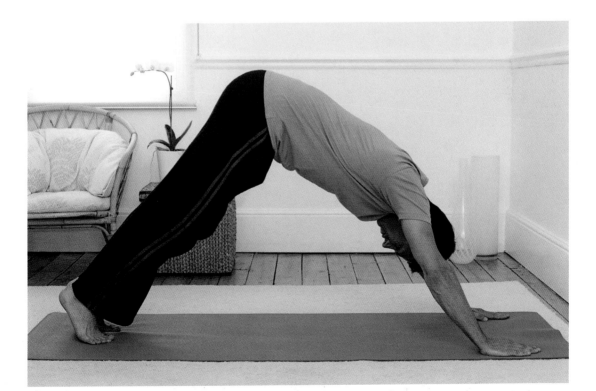

Lying Back and Leg Stretch

What it does

Stretches and strengthens the back muscles

Helps to ease tension in the back

Tones the abdominal muscles, which give support to the back

Stretches and strengthens the leg muscles, which are secondary back supports

How to do it

1 Lie on your back with your legs stretched out in front. Relax your arms at your sides. Breathe regularly.

2 Bend your right knee and bring it towards your chest. Tuck the fingers of your right hand under the toes. Do the same with the left knee and fingers.

3 Holding the toes securely, carefully raise and straighten your legs as much as you can with absolute comfort. Be careful not to strain.

4 Hold the posture for five or more seconds while breathing regularly.

5 Release your hold on the toes and carefully lower one leg at a time to resume your starting position. Rest briefly.

6 You may repeat the exercise (steps 2 to 5) once or twice.

7 Stretch out your legs and rest.

Alternative Lying Back and Leg Stretch

How to do it

1 Vary the basic exercise above by carefully spreading your legs apart to their comfortable limit.

2 Hold the spread-legs posture for five or more seconds.

3 Carefully resume your starting position. Rest briefly.

4 You may repeat the exercise once or twice.

5 Stretch out your legs and rest.

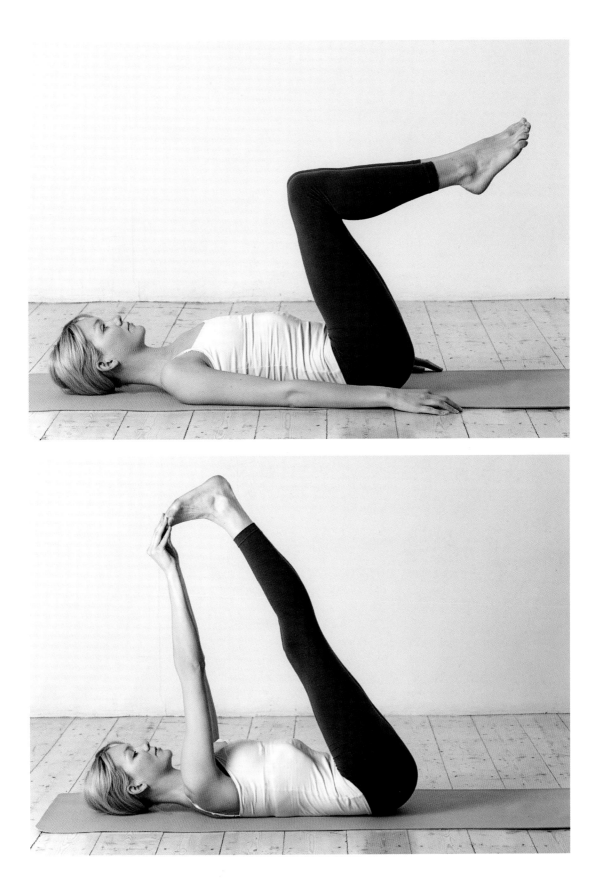

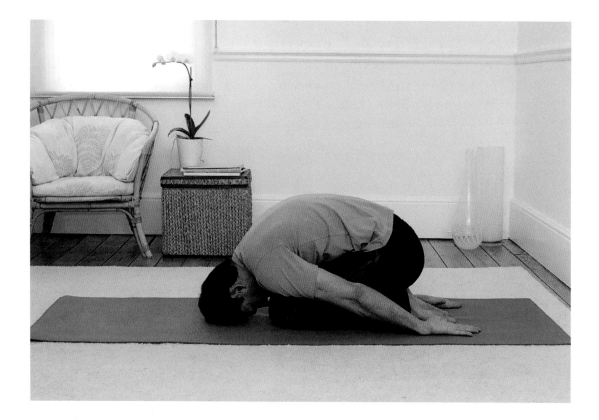

Crouching (Prayer) Posture

What it does

Gives a beneficial stretch to the back muscles

Wonderfully relaxing for the back

Helps to relieve pressure on spinal discs by widening the spaces between the vertebrae, where the discs are located

Eases pressure on nerves branching from the spine and so helps to relieve pain

Helps to keep the spine flexible

How to do it

1 Sit on your heels on a mat, Japanese style. Breathe regularly.

2 Slowly bend forwards and rest your head on the mat. Relax your arms at your sides.

3 Stay in this posture for five to twenty seconds or longer.

4 Slowly resume your starting position.

NOTES

In step 2 above, you may rest your head on a small pillow or cushion. You may also try doing this exercise with a bolster between your knees, and your arms resting at the sides of it.

Alternative healing back sequence

This sequence is probably a little more challenging than the first one and offers some variety. Start with the warm ups on pages 62–73. Then follow with the exercises below.

Prone Leg Raise

What it does

Strengthens the back muscles

Stretches and strengthens the abdominal muscles, which give support to the back muscles

Strengthens the leg muscles, which are secondary back supports

How to do it

1 Lie on your abdomen. Rest your chin on the mat. Keep your legs close together and your arms on the mat, straight and close to your sides. Breathe regularly.

2 On an exhalation, slowly raise one straight leg as high as you comfortably can. Hold the raised-leg posture for five or more seconds while breathing regularly.

3 Carefully lower your leg and rest briefly.

4 Repeat the exercise (steps 2 to 4) with the other leg. Rest.

5 You may repeat the sequence (steps 2 to 4) once or twice.

CAUTION
Omit this exercise if you are pregnant, or if you have a hernia or a heart disorder.

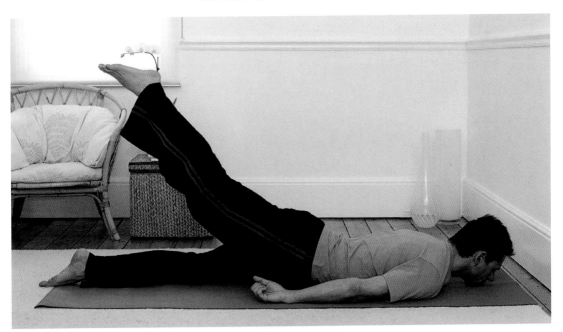

Back Arch

What it does

Helps to keep the spine flexible

Strengthens neck and back muscles

Enhances spinal circulation

How to do it

1 Lie on your abdomen. Rest your forehead on the mat. Rest your palms under your shoulders. Breathe regularly.

2 Inhale and slowly and carefully begin to arch your spine backwards, from neck to chest. Keep your hips on the mat.

3 Hold the posture for five or more seconds while breathing regularly.

4 Very slowly and carefully, return to your starting position in reverse order. Rest briefly, with your head turned to the side and arms relaxed beside you.

5 You may repeat the exercise (steps 1 to 4) once or twice.

CAUTION

Omit this exercise if you are pregnant, or if you have a hernia or neck pain.

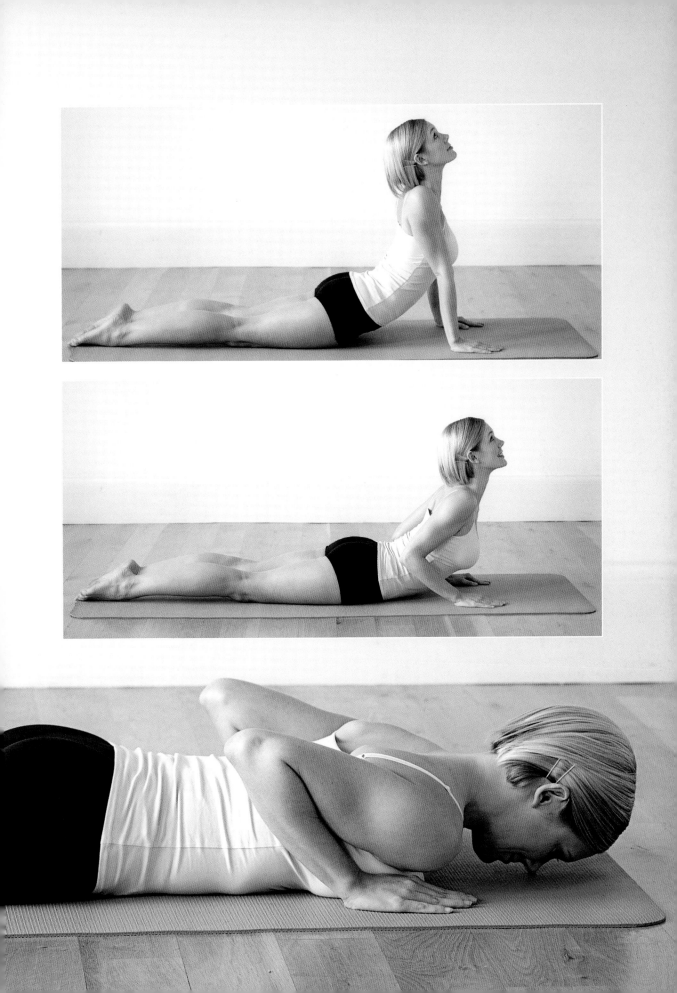

Arm and Leg Lift

What it does

Strengthens the back muscles

Stretches and strengthens the leg muscles, which are secondary back supports

Stretches and strengthens the abdominal muscles, which give reinforcement to the back

How to do it

1 Start in an all-fours position, on your hands and knees. Breathe regularly.

2 Inhale and lift your left arm and right leg and fully stretch them.

3 Hold the raised-limbs posture for five or more seconds while breathing regularly.

4 Resume your starting position.

5 Repeat the exercise (steps 2 to 4) with your right arm and left leg. Rest briefly.

6 Repeat the entire sequence (steps 2 to 5) once or twice. Rest.

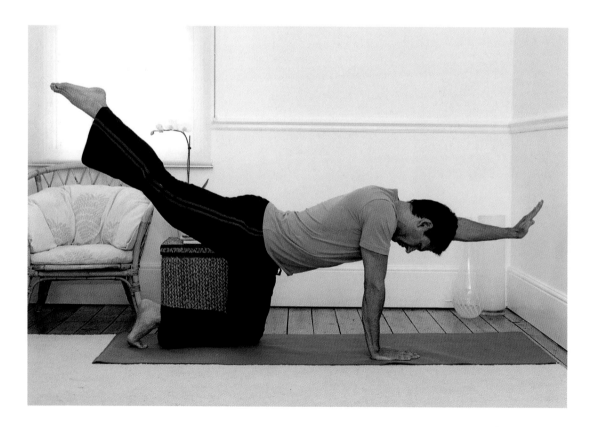

Crouching (Prayer) Posture (see also page 90)

What it does

Gives a beneficial stretch to the back muscles

Wonderfully relaxing for the back

Helps to relieve pressure on spinal discs by widening the spaces between the vertebrae, where the discs are located

Eases pressure on nerves branching from the spine and so helps to relieve pain

Helps to keep the spine flexible

How to do it

1 Sit on your heels on a mat, Japanese style. Breathe regularly.

2 Slowly bend forwards and rest your head on the mat. Relax your arms at your sides.

3 Stay in this posture for five to twenty seconds or longer.

4 Slowly resume your starting position.

NOTES

In step 2 above, you may rest your head on a small pillow or cushion. You may also try doing this exercise with a bolster between your knees, and your arms resting at the sides of it.

VARIATION

Instead of resting your arms at your sides, as in step 2 above, stretch them ahead of you and rest them on the mat.

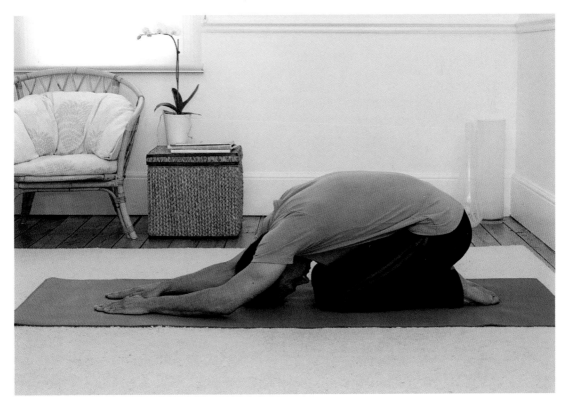

Spinal Twist

What it does

Allows maximum torsion (twisting) of the spine to both sides and so provides a gentle, therapeutic massage to nerves branching from the spinal column

Helps to keep the spine flexible

Tones the lower back muscles

Tones the transverse and oblique abdominal muscles (page 13)

Enhances spinal circulation

How to do it

1 Sit tall with your legs stretched out in front. Breathe regularly.

2 Bend your right leg and rest the foot on the mat outside the left knee.

3 Exhale and smoothly swivel your upper body to the right, as far as you comfortably can.

4 Look over your right shoulder. Rest one or both hands on the mat on your right.

5 Hold the twist for five or more seconds while breathing regularly.

6 Inhale and slowly resume your starting position. Rest briefly.

7 Repeat the exercise (steps 2 to 5) on the other side (substitute the word 'left' for 'right' and vice versa).

8 Repeat the entire exercise (steps 2 to 6) once or twice. Rest.

See also page 97.

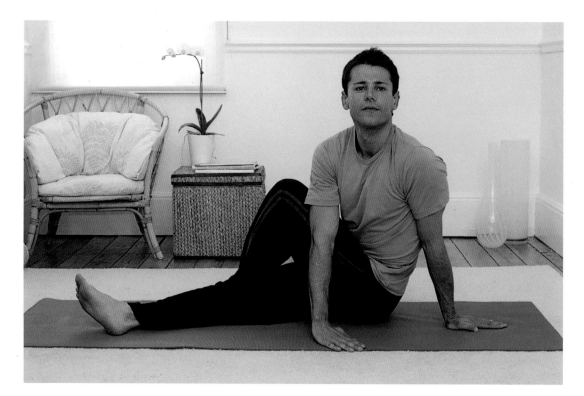

Sideways Arch

What it does
Strengthens the back muscles

Helps to keep the spine flexible

Conditions abdominal muscles, which are often under-exercised, to provide reinforcement for back muscles

Facilitates efficient breathing, which can be restricted in some spinal disorders (see ankylosing spondylitis on page 122)

How to do it

1 Stand tall with your feet close together and arms at your sides. Breathe regularly.

2 Inhale and stretch your arms overhead. Keep them close to your ears and bring the palms together if you can.

3 Exhale and smoothly bend your upper torso to one side, as far as you comfortably can.

4 Hold this sideways arch for five or more seconds while breathing regularly.

5 Inhale and resume your starting position. Rest briefly.

6 Repeat the exercise (steps 2 to 5) on the other side.

7 Repeat the entire exercise (steps 2 to 6) once or twice. Rest.

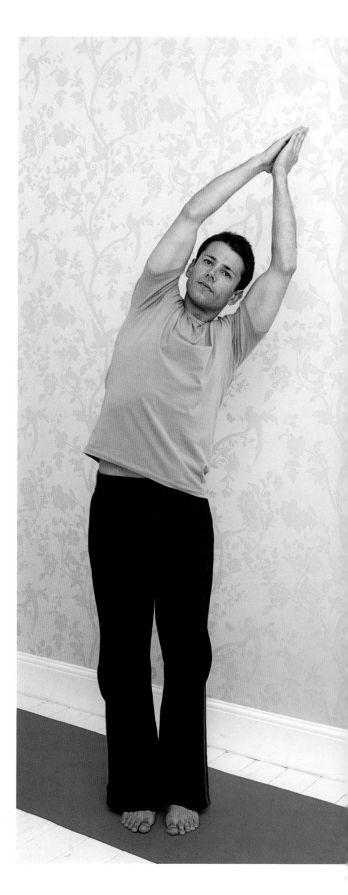

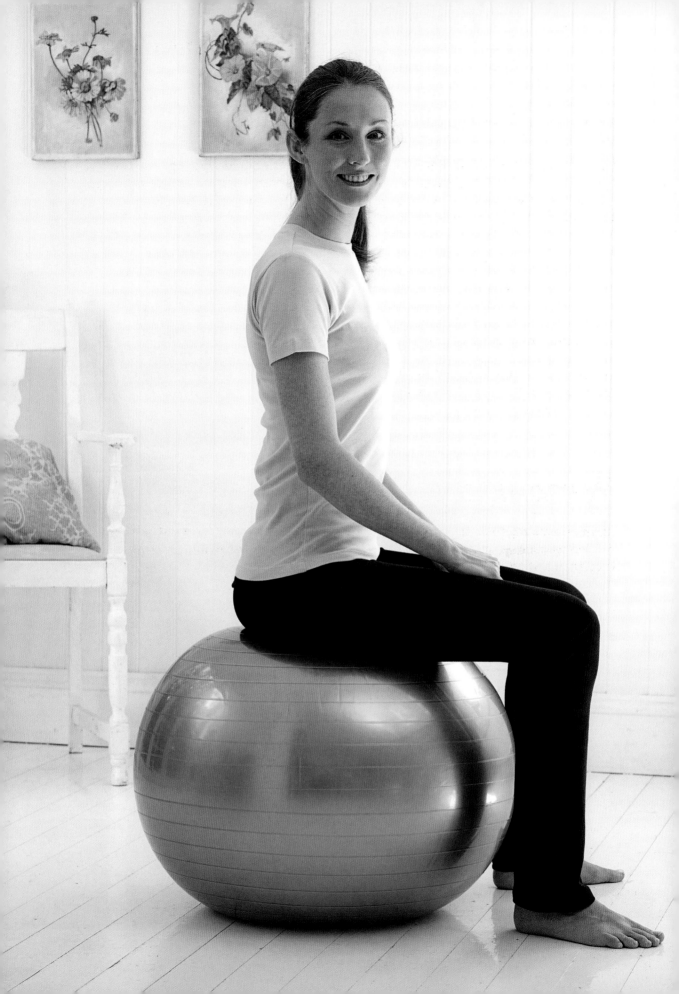

Back on the ball

The Swiss ball (which is known by various other names, including exercise, fitness and stability ball) has long been used by physiotherapists for rehabilitation and other therapeutic purposes. Its effectiveness lies, surprisingly, in its instability: your muscles have to work to keep both the ball and your body stable.

Ball benefits

Exercises ordinarily under-utilised muscles to make them more efficient.

Improves posture.

Strengthens postural muscles (those of the back, abdomen and legs).

Lessens fatigue.

Improves concentration and so reduces the risk of inadvertent injury.

Gives support to body parts during rehabilitation exercise, after injury or illness and decreases pain.

Warm ups

Before attempting to do the main Swiss Ball exercises, it's important to spend at least five minutes warming up to reduce stiffness, slightly increase body temperature, enhance circulation and prevent pulls and strains.

When and how

Successful ball work partly depends on choosing a ball that's right for you. A simple guide is that when you sit on the ball, with your feet flat on the floor, your thighs should be parallel to the floor and your hip and knee joints should each form a 90-degree angle. Personnel at the store where you purchase your ball can be helpful, and the manufacturers' guidelines are generally easy to follow.

Sit tall on the centre of the ball.

Rest your feet flat on the floor, shoulders' width apart.

Rest your hands on your thighs or on the sides of the ball.

Secure in this position, proceed to do the Neck Stretches (page 65) and Shoulder Rolls (page 62). Follow these with Hip Circles (page 100).

Hip Circles

What they do

Keep the joints of the lower spine freely moving

Contribute to flexibility of the lower spine

Tone the lower back and abdominal muscles

How to do them

1 Sit on the ball and rotate your hips as if drawing smooth imaginary circles: shift your weight to one 'sitting bone' (under the buttock), then tilt your pelvis backwards. Shift your weight to the other sitting bone and complete the circle by tilting the pelvis forwards to complete one rotation.

2 Repeat the exercise twice in the same direction.

3 Repeat the exercise twice in the opposite direction.

NOTE

Keep your upper body as still as you can and breathe regularly while doing the Hip Circles.

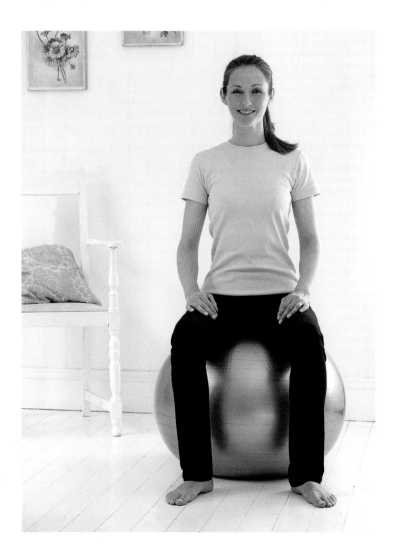

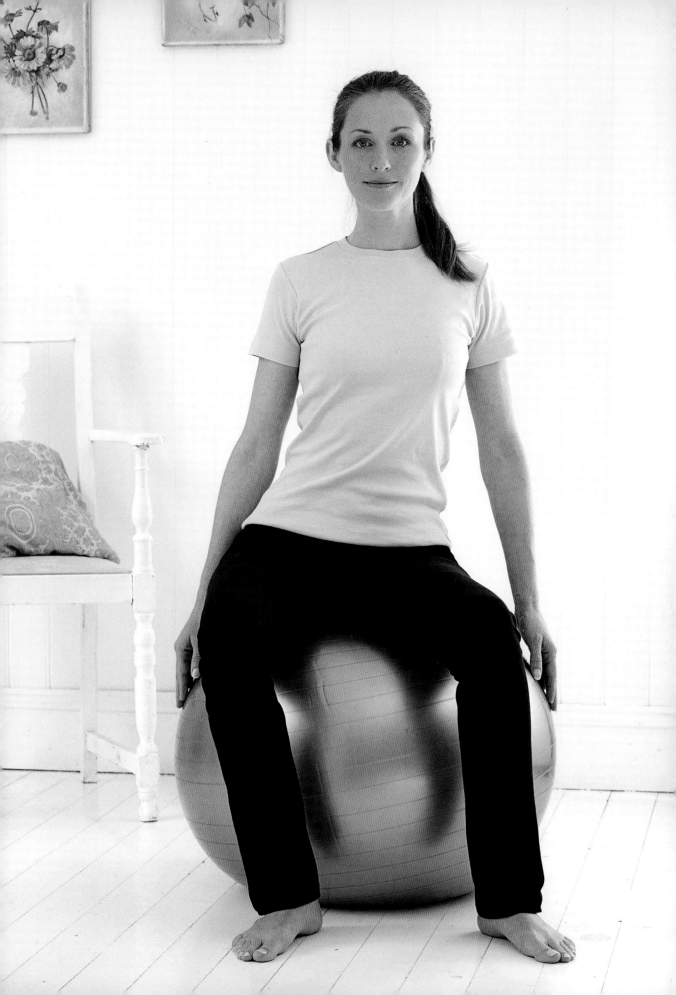

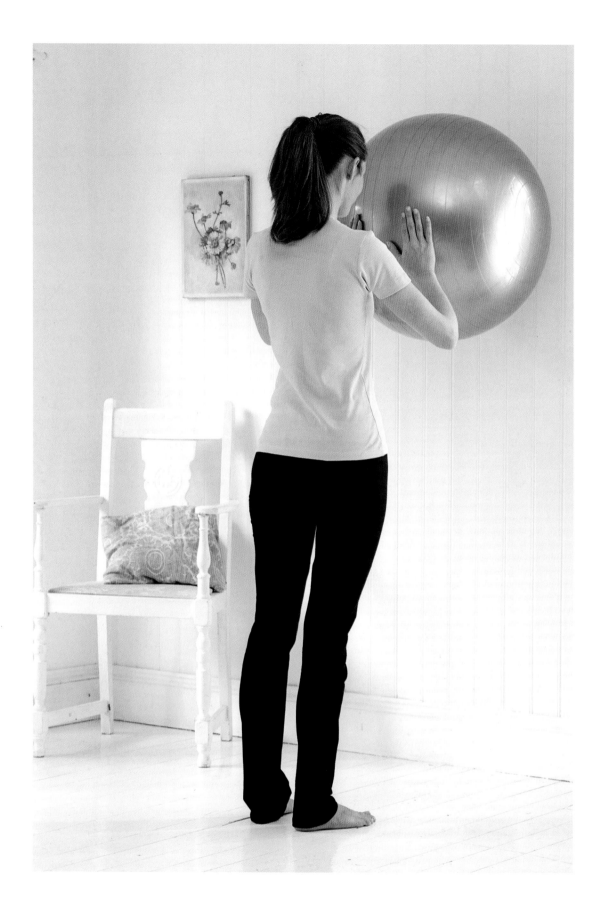

Swiss ball exercises

The following exercises have been specially chosen for their excellent ability, with regular practice, to help keep the spine flexible, to tone and strengthen the postural muscles (those of the neck, back, abdomen and legs), and to facilitate breathing, through which all tissues receive oxygen.

Wall Crawl

What it does

Tones and strengthens muscles of the upper back and chest

Promotes efficient breathing, for better delivery of oxygen to the body's tissues

Useful in conditions such as ankylosing spondylitis (page 122) where ribcage expansion and unrestricted breathing may be compromised

How to do it

1 Stand facing a wall. Place a ball between your upper body and the wall.

2 Rest a hand securely on each side of the ball, as if preparing to push it upwards. Breathe regularly.

3 Use both hands for the initial upward roll of the ball, then use alternate hands to continue, until your arms are fully but comfortably stretched.

4 Hold the stretch for five or more seconds while breathing regularly.

5 Roll the ball downwards to the starting position.

6 Repeat the exercise twice. Remove the ball. Rest.

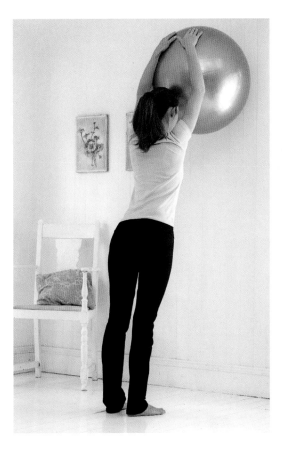

Wall Squat

What it does

Tones and strengthens back and abdominal muscles

Tones and strengthens leg muscles, which are secondary back supports

See also Squatting Posture (page 86)

How to do it

1 Stand tall with a ball placed securely between your back and wall. Breathe regularly.

2 Slowly bend your knees as if preparing to sit down, until your thighs are roughly parallel to the floor, if you can.

3 Hold the posture for five seconds or more while breathing regularly.

4 Slowly return to a standing position.

5 Repeat the exercise (steps 2 to 4) twice. Rest.

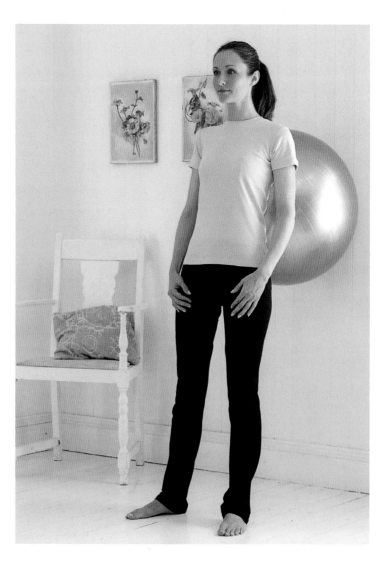

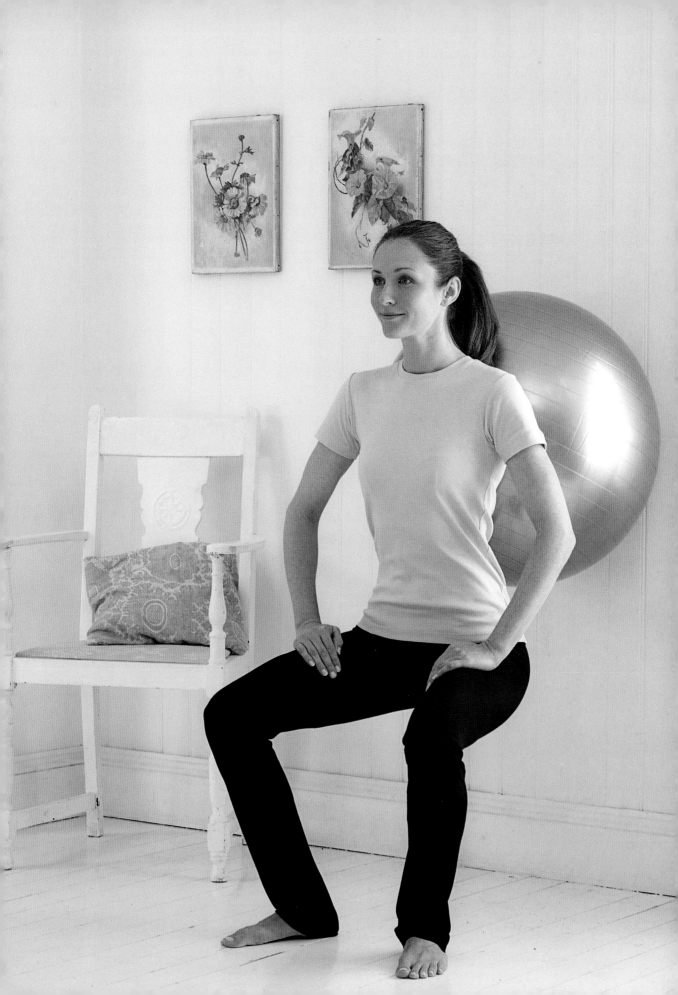

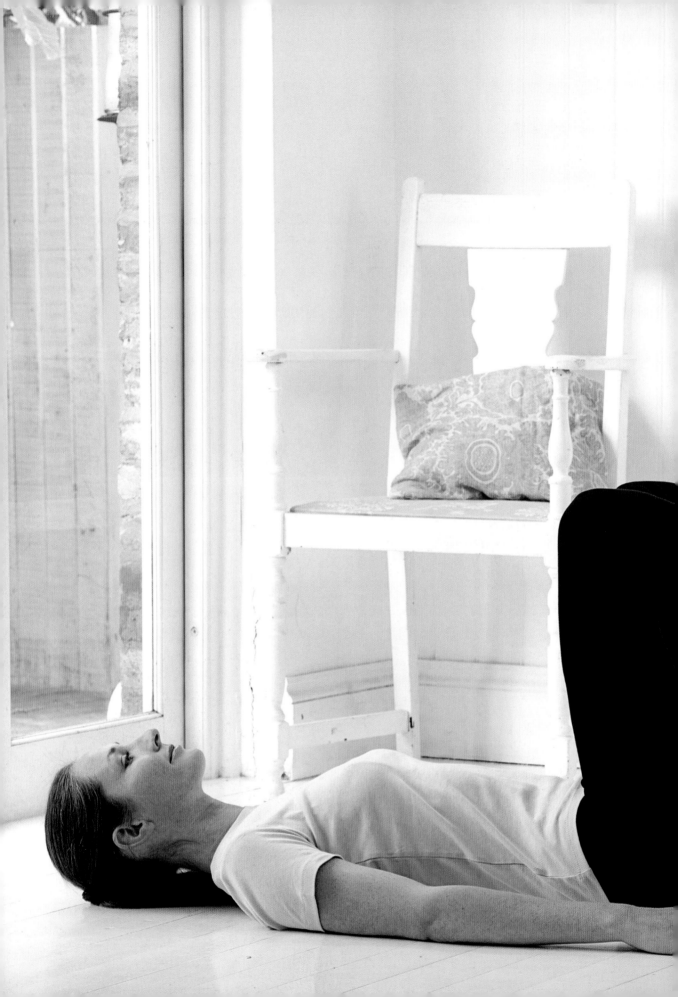

Swiss Ball Bridge

What it does

Tones the muscles of the back

Helps to keep the spine flexible

Tones abdominal muscles, which provide reinforcement for the back

Strengthens and tones the leg muscles, which are secondary back supports

How to do it

1 Lie on your back, with your knees bent and feet resting on a ball. Breathe regularly.

2 On an inhalation, slowly, carefully and with control, raise your torso from hips to upper back. Stay fully focused in order to keep the ball stable.

3 When you have reached your comfortable limit, hold the posture for five or more seconds while breathing regularly.

4 To return to your starting position, slowly and with control lower your torso from top to bottom. Put your feet on the mat and stretch out your legs and rest.

5 You may repeat the exercise (steps 2 to 4) once or twice.

Supine Hamstring Stretch

What it does

Strengthens the muscles of the back

Strengthens the abdominal muscles, which give reinforcement to the back

Helps to maintain the elasticity of the hamstrings: when these muscles shorten, they affect the angle of pelvic tilt and so influence posture

How to do it

1 Lie on your back facing a wall, with your bottom close to it and your feet resting against it. Relax your arms at your sides and breathe regularly.

2 Bend your knees and place a ball securely between your feet and the wall.

3 Slowly and attentively straighten your legs to their comfortable limit. As you do so, the ball will roll up the wall.

4 Hold the leg stretch for five or more seconds while breathing regularly.

5 Bend your legs to resume your starting position (step 2). As you do so, the ball will roll down the wall.

6 You may repeat the exercise (steps 2 to 5) once or twice.

7 Put the ball aside and turn on your side to get up safely (page 74). Rest.

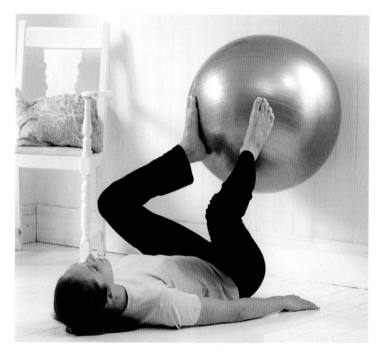

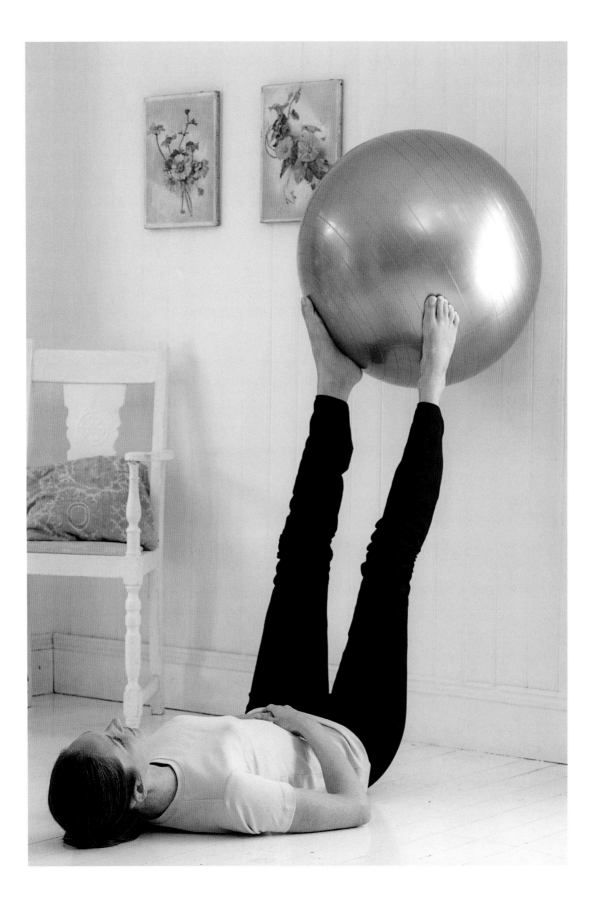

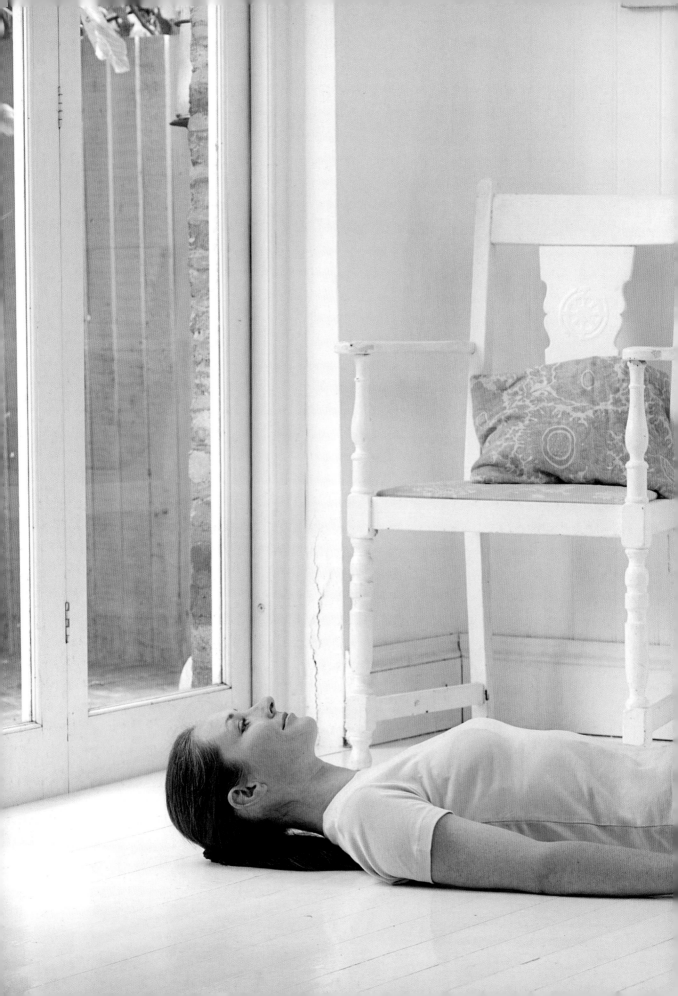

Other ways to use the ball

As a chair

At a desk, a computer or other keyboard or while watching television, for short periods. This trains you in 'active sitting' and subtly exercises postural muscles and improves balance.

As a footstool

Sit on a chair or couch and elevate your legs by resting your feet on a ball. This relaxes back muscles and lessens fatigue.

As a postural aid

Lie on a carpeted floor and rest your feet on a ball, instead of a padded chair seat (as described on page 44).

Cooling down

Cooling down after exercise allows your cardiovascular (heart and blood vessel) system to return to natural functioning in a gradual way. This prevents dizziness and lightheadedness, which can signal a sudden drop in blood pressure. Cooling down exercises also provide a chance for static muscle stretching.

The following exercises, which were described on pages 62–73, are suitable for cool-downs. Do them very slowly and attentively, and in synchronisation with regular breathing. To avoid back strain, maintain good posture.

- Neck Stretches
- Shoulder Rolls
- Pelvic Tilt
- Reclining Twist
- The alternative to the Spinal Roll (Pelvic Tilt on all fours)

You may, in addition, add the All-Body Stretch opposite.

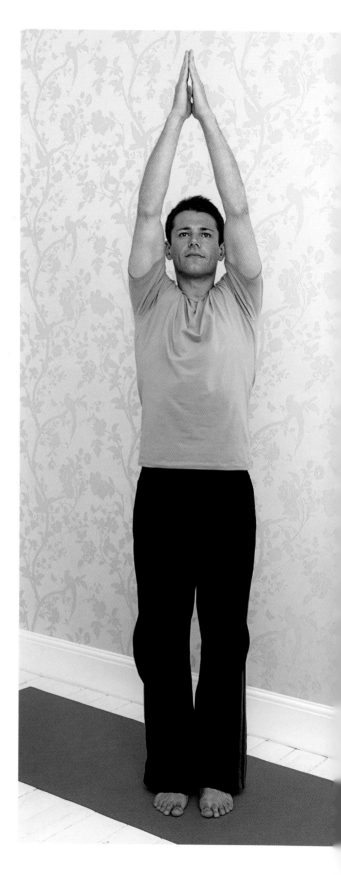

All-Body Stretch

What it does

Relaxes tense abdominal muscles

Allows for maximum stretching of the body

Helps to counteract faulty postures

How to do it

1 Lie on your back with legs straight in front and arms at your sides. Breathe regularly.

2 Inhale and stretch your arms straight overhead. Simultaneously stretch your legs, bring your toes towards you and push your heels away.

3 Hold the all-body stretch for five or more seconds while breathing regularly.

4 Exhale, release the stretch and resume your starting position. Rest briefly and breathe regularly.

5 Repeat the exercise (steps 2 to 4) once or twice. Rest.

Alternative All-Body Stretch

How to do it

1 Stand tall with your weight equally distributed between your feet and your arms relaxed at your sides. Breathe regularly.

2 Inhale and fully stretch your arms overhead. Bring your palms together if you can. Hold the stretch for five or more seconds while breathing regularly.

3 Exhale and lower your arms.

4 You may repeat the exercise (steps 2 and 3) once or twice. Rest.

Ailments and Healing Options

Whenever a health disorder occurs, it seldom affects only one part of the body. Pain felt in a leg, for example, may originate from pressure on a spinal nerve by a narrowed spinal canal. This, in turn, could be the result of disc herniation.

For convenient reading and reference, however, this chapter has been organised into component categories and is based on the format used in the chapter on what can go wrong.

Spinal cord and nerves

The spinal cord, which is an extension of the brain, occupies the spinal canal within the vertebral column. Anything that places pressure on the tissues or causes injury can produce bothersome symptoms.

Sciatica

Sciatica is an inflammation of the sciatic nerve along its course down the back of the thigh and lower leg.

Symptoms

Symptoms of sciatica may worsen at night or with impending stormy weather, and may last from a few days to several months. They include:

- Mild to severe back pain radiating to the buttock and thigh, worsened by coughing, sneezing or bending
- Numbness or tingling in the lower leg
- Muscle weakness in the buttock, thigh, lower leg or foot

Causes

Among the causes contributing to sciatica are:

- Trauma to or compression of the sciatic nerve or its roots, such as that produced by a herniated intervertebral disc
- Inflammation of the sciatic nerve, caused by an infection for example
- Pain referred to the nerve from another part of the body

Increasing the risk of developing sciatica are: a back injury, a herniated disc, being overweight, a sedentary lifestyle and incorrect body mechanics.

Prevention

- Regular exercise, with emphasis on strengthening the muscles of the back, abdomen and legs.
- Good habits of posture and body mechanics
- Avoiding being overweight

Treatments

The following are some choices of treatment for sciatica, depending on the symptoms:

- Reduced activity, rather than bed rest, to ease

pressure on the nerve and facilitate healing
- Application of heat, such as a heating pad or soaking in a hot bath, to ease pain and muscle spasm
- Analgesic (pain-relieving) or anti-inflammatory medication such as NSAIDs
- Surgery, as in some cases of a herniated disc

Alternative treatments:

- Physiotherapy, such as ultrasound, applications of cold, hydrotherapy and electrical nerve stimulation
- Acupuncture
- Chiropractic (except in cases of a herniated disc)

Spinal stenosis

The word stenosis comes from Greek and means narrow. Spinal stenosis is a narrowing of the spinal canal, which reduces the space available to the spinal cord and nerves.

Those most at risk of developing this condition are: the elderly, people with a herniated disc, spinal tumour, infection or vertebral fracture, and those who are overweight or inactive.

Symptoms

Symptoms of spinal stenosis include:

- Pain in the buttocks and low back, which may radiate to one or both legs
- Numbness in the legs, which eases with rest and bending forwards and worsens with activity
- Weakness and impaired balance
- A foot-slapping gait

Causes

Among the conditions that can lead to spinal stenosis:

- Degenerative arthritis
- Spondylolisthesis (page 124)

- Trauma,
- Bone disease
- Genetic factors

Prevention

Two of the best measures for helping to avert spinal stenosis are:

- Taking steps to improve posture and body mechanics (pages 42–55)
- Regularly engaging in simple stretching and strengthening exercises

Additional measures include:

- Controlling your body weight with sensible eating
- Keeping active
- Not smoking (smoking accelerates disc degeneration because it limits blood supply, and it also increases the risk of disc herniation)

Treatments

NSAIDs are generally useful for reducing inflammation and discomfort.

Other therapeutic measures to consider are applications of heat or cold, and low-impact exercises such as swimming (but first check with your doctor).

For those to whom the above treatments bring no relief, or whose functioning becomes increasingly impaired, injection therapy (page 37) or decompression surgery (page 39) may be worth considering.

Alternative treatments:

Although it will not correct the underlying cause, acupuncture may be a useful alternative to other treatments for relieving pain.

Other therapies to try include: ultrasound, diathermy, TENS and massage.

Cauda Equina Syndrome

The cauda equina is the terminal portion of the spinal cord (page 12). Cauda Equina Syndrome consists of a set of symptoms that characterise a particular disorder.

Symptoms

- Inability to pass urine
- Leaking from a full bladder
- Progressive loss of feeling between the legs
- Progressive loss of power and feeling in both legs

Causes and treatment

Cauda Equina Syndrome is a result of significant pressure on the structures within the spinal canal. This is a red flag condition (page 16), which, because of its serious nature, requires immediate medical attention and possible decompression surgery.

Bones

Thirty-three bones form the spine, or vertebral column. Any of these can be damaged by trauma or other forces, including infection, degenerative changes or wear and tear over time.

Fractures

A fracture, in the simplest of terms, is a broken bone.

Symptoms

Among the symptoms of a fractured spinal bone, or vertebra, are:

- Back pain, sometimes radiating to the buttocks
- Rapidly occurring pain
- Pain while resting

Causes

Causes of a fractured vertebra include:

- Trauma, as in a car accident, a sports event or a blow to the back
- Disease, as from osteoporosis and metastases (spread) from cancer (for example, in the breast or prostate gland)
- Use of steroids to treat inflammatory disorders such as arthritis, for example.

Prevention

If the fracture is due to osteoporosis, certain precautionary measures can be taken to delay its onset or avert its occurrence (see opposite). The chances of fracture from a fall can be lessened by regular exercises that improve balance and coordination and by prudent safety measures, which include sensible footwear and non-skid surfaces in bathtubs and on stairs.

Emergency alert

Back pain and associated symptoms occurring after a fall or other accident could indicate serious damage and should be treated as an emergency. The following precautions should be taken:

- Discourage the injured person from moving
- Do not move the injured person
- Call your medical emergency service for assistance (a specially trained team will appropriately mobilise the injured individual's spine and safely transfer him or her to a treatment facility)

Treating vertebral compression fractures

The following are possible measures for treating compression fractures, depending on their cause:

- An extension brace, to be worn for about three or four months, with periodic X-rays taken to assess healing or deformity
- Good posture when lying down (page 44), avoiding the prone position
- Possibly taking nutritional supplements to promote bone health, such as calcium and magnesium, boron, zinc and vitamin D (check with a qualified nutrition specialist)
- Avoiding alcoholic, caffeinated and carbonated drinks, which can detract from bone health
- Analgesics to relieve pain, and anti-inflammatory drugs to counteract inflammation
- Fairly rapid but graduated mobilisation following impaired functioning, to build strength and confidence (a physiotherapist may be helpful)
- Appropriate treatment if osteoporosis is the cause of fracture (see opposite)

Surgical treatments

When less invasive treatments fail to bring the desired results, surgery may become necessary. Operations include vertebroplasty and kyphoplasty (page 39).

Osteoporosis

Osteoporosis, which literally means 'porous bones', describes a disease process in which bones become brittle and weak and prone to fractures. The most serious loss of bone integrity occurs in the spine and femur (thigh bone). Once weakened, the vertebrae can become easily compressed by the weight of the body itself. When this happens, it can reduce your height by several inches/centimetres.

Symptoms

Difficulty in bending forwards and back pain are two symptoms that suggest osteoporosis. As the disease process advances, height may be noticeably decreased, and sometimes a kyphosis (dowager's hump) may develop. If the bones of the ribcage are involved, it may affect efficient breathing.

Causes

Osteoporosis mostly affects post-menopausal women and, to a lesser extent, sedentary men. It can also occur among young women who drastically limit their food intake to become or stay thin: nutrients crucial to the health and strength of bones, such as calcium, vitamin D, boron and zinc, become inadequate.

Bone integrity can also be compromised by the frequent use of antacids (substances that neutralise acid) containing aluminium, since they accelerate the excretion of calcium. Some diuretics (water pills), which promote calcium loss, and some laxatives, especially mineral oil, if used frequently, can deplete supplies of important mineral and vitamins. In addition, steroids, sometimes administered in the treatment of inflammatory diseases such as arthritis, may inhibit bone formation and calcium absorption.

Prevention

Preventive measures should begin in early adulthood to build bone mass and strength. This includes a diet rich in bone-building nutrients such as calcium, vitamin D, zinc and boron and regular weight-bearing exercise such as walking, dancing and stair-climbing.

It would be prudent, in addition, to avoid smoking, which is believed to be toxic to bone, and to keep consumption of alcohol, caffeinated beverages and carbonated drinks low, since these are thought to deplete the body of essential nutrients. Avoid regular use of antacids containing aluminium, which tend to promote bone loss.

Learn and habitually practise stress-management techniques to help keep the level of cortisol (stress hormone) low.

Treatments

Once osteoporosis has occurred, treatments tend to produce less than ideal results. Nevertheless, ensuring the intake of essential nutrients, such as those already mentioned above, is useful in slowing down the progression of bone loss. Best among the food sources of such nutrients are: green leafy vegetables, dairy and soybean products and whole grains. Nutritional supplements may also be helpful, but first check with your doctor or other qualified health professional.

Post-menopausal women should discuss hormone replacement therapy with their doctor, and possibly also other medicines to increase bone mass and decrease bone loss.

Regular exercise is essential not only in helping to prevent osteoporosis but also to slow down its progression. Caution is needed, however, in attempting to do flexion exercises (forward-bending movements) if the vertebrae are involved. Please check with your doctor or physiotherapist. Exercises to improve coordination and balance are important, as they can help to prevent falls and possible resulting fracture.

Stress management strategies should be part of daily life, as mentioned above.

Medicines used to treat osteoporosis include:

- Bisphosphonates, which reduce bone resorption (loss of bone substance), and which may also increase the activity of bone-building cells (osteoblasts)
- SERM (Selective Estrogen Receptor Modulations), which reduce bone resorption, but which should be given only post-menopausally
- Calcitonin to reduce bone resorption and possibly increase bone-building cells, and which may also be useful in relieving pain

- Teriparatide (Forteo), an injectable hormone derived from the parathyroid glands (which are involved in calcium metabolism), which helps to increase bone formation
- Hormone replacement therapy may be considered to increase osteoblast activity and reduce bone resorption, but it may not be appropriate for all women. It should be carefully discussed with your doctor, as it has the potential to produce some adverse effects.

- Non-prescription analgesics such as aspirin and paracetamol can provide pain relief.

Alternative treatments:
- Local applications of heat, such as a heating pad
- Nutritional therapy
- T'ai Chi
- Yoga

Joints

Joints are connections between bones. Between every two vertebrae are joints formed by smooth cartilage and strengthened by ligaments that run behind and in front of the vertebral bodies throughout the entire length of the spine. In addition, there are facet joints at the back of the vertebrae (page 12). Like joints elsewhere in the body, spinal joints are vulnerable to injury by infection or tumour, by degenerative processes, or by trauma.

Osteoarthritis (OA)

Known also as non-inflammatory arthritis or degenerative joint disease, osteoarthritis is the most common type of arthritis and tends to occur in older individuals. It affects the smooth cartilage covering the ends of bones where they form joints. It can also involve the underlying bone and surrounding tissues and other spinal components, such as discs and ligaments.

Although inflammation is not typical of OA, changes in the joints may sometimes produce a local inflammatory response.

Symptoms

Stiffness and back pain, which may worsen with extension (bending backwards), could be an indication of spinal osteoarthritis. The pain, however, is rarely disabling.

OA in the low back can lead to a narrowing of the spinal canal (see stenosis, page 116) or to slippage of a vertebra (see spondylolisthesis, page 000) and produce other symptoms, including pain that radiates to, and numbness and weakness in, the legs.

Causes

OA can develop following trauma or other injury, an inflammatory joint disease, or repetitive strain related to your occupation or sports activities.

Prevention

To help prevent the occurrence or progression of OA:
- Maintain good general health, with attention to a diet rich in essential minerals and vitamins
- Avoid being overweight
- Exercise daily to maintain spinal strength and flexibility
- Practise good posture and body mechanics to minimise stress on spinal structures

Treatments

Among the treatment choices for dealing with OA are:
- Heat, through local application such as a heat pack, by immersion in a whirlpool bath, or with a warm shower
- Hands-on treatments such as Shiatsu or other form of massage (inflamed areas should not be massaged, however)

- Non-prescription analgesics such as paracetamol
- Topical application of capsicum cream. (Capsicum is found in chilli, red and cayenne peppers and has anti-inflammatory properties.)
- Stretching and strengthening exercises
- Injection therapy (page 37) or surgery where applicable

Alternative treatments:
- Acupuncture for pain relief
- Herbal medicine, including sources of essential fatty acids (EFAs, see below) to help reduce inflammation
- Nutritional therapy, which includes supplements of nutrients such as vitamins C, D and E, and also of glucosamine (a cartilage-building material and a component of synovial fluid) and chondroitin (a vital part of the 'glue' that maintains the integrity of joint cartilage)
- Yoga and T'ai Chi
- Relaxation techniques

EFAs are called 'essential' because the body must have them to carry out certain vital functions. But since the body cannot make them, they have to be provided by food. Food sources of EFAs include flax seeds, soy beans and walnuts, and oils from these; dark green leaves; and cold-water fish such as salmon, sardines and trout. Supplementary sources of EFAs include oils from blackcurrants, borage and evening primrose.

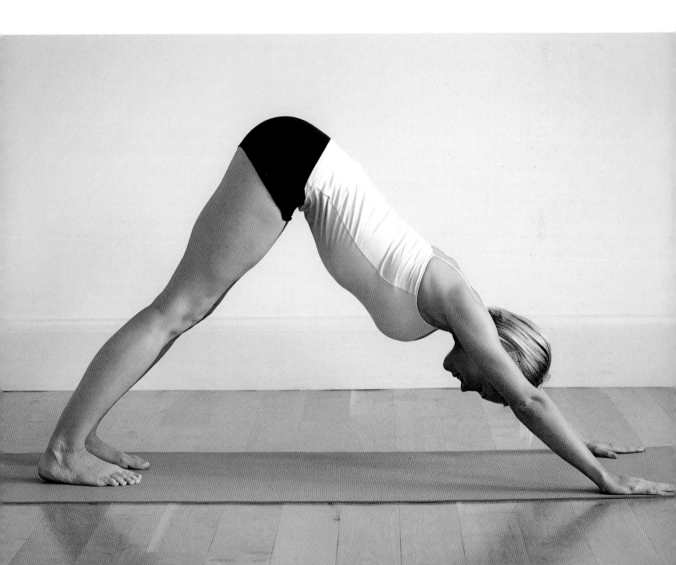

Rheumatoid arthritis (RA)

Rheumatoid arthritis is an inflammatory type of arthritis that affects connective tissue, most notably synovial joints (which contain a lubricating fluid to facilitate movement). Its incidence is two times higher in women than in men, until the age of 65 years, when both are almost equally affected.

Symptoms

For most RA sufferers, the condition first produces fatigue and general malaise. Stiffness is noticeable after inactivity, especially after sleeping at night. With progression of the disease, loss of function increases.

Although RA affects mostly the hands and feet, it also occurs not infrequently in the cervical spine. If neck involvement is severe, spinal cord compression may result and surgery may become necessary.

RA can develop in the low back also, where it can affect facet joints, ligaments and other adjacent structures and produce pain.

Causes

RA was once believed to be an autoimmune disease, in which the body literally turns against itself, but this is currently in question.

There appears to be a genetic predisposition to RA, and hormonal fluctuations seem to play a part also. For example, symptoms tend to abate during the last trimester of pregnancy but flare up following childbirth. Infection can also be a contributing cause.

Prevention

Preventive measures to take against RA include joint protection and regular appropriate exercise to help to maintain function. Joint protection consists essentially of learning and practising good habits of posture and body mechanics and taking breaks from prolonged or repetitive activity to do simple stretching exercises. Regularly engaging in appropriate exercises is one key to maintaining function and preventing disability. A physiotherapist or other qualified professional can help you. The therapist can also be of assistance in the safe use of mobility aids such as walkers.

Treatments

Treatments for people with RA aim to relieve pain, reduce inflammation, protect joint surfaces and maintain function. In addition to relieving pain and reducing inflammation, anti-inflammatory medications are also used to help prevent the progression of RA from a localised area to other body parts. These drugs include aspirin, NSAIDs such as ibuprofen and naproxen to decrease pain and swelling, short-term use of glucocorticoids such as prednisone and cortisone, and slow-acting anti-rheumatic drugs.

Alternative treatments:

- Local applications of heat
- Massage therapy
- Nutritional supplements including EFAs (essential fatty acids, see page 121), glucosamine sulphate and chondroitin sulphate (see Osteoarthritis, page 120)
- T'ai Chi
- Yoga
- Relaxation techniques

Ankylosing spondylitis (AS)

Ankylosing spondylitis is a chronic, progressive inflammation of the spine and sacroiliac joints. It affects mostly males, usually before the age of 40 years. Its origin is unknown, but a strong hereditary tendency is suspected.

Symptoms

The most common symptom of AS is pain in the low back and upper buttocks, which comes on gradually and persists for at least three months. It worsens with rest and eases with graduated activity. The pain can also radiate to the upper back and sometimes to the breastbone. Stiffness, which is more noticeable after a night's sleep, is another symptom.

AS can also affect other body tissues, including those of the heart, lungs, kidneys and eyes, spinal ligaments and tendons, sacroiliac joints and the joints between the ribs and vertebrae, which can cause breathing difficulties.

Other manifestations of AS include general malaise and weight loss and, as the disorder

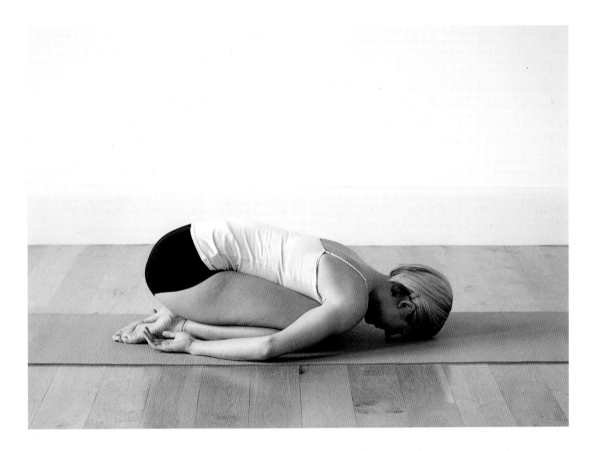

progresses, a fusing together of the vertebrae, increased arching of the upper back and rigidity of the neck.

Causes

The cause of AS is not known with certainty, but heredity and infection are thought to be implicated.

Treatments

There appear to be no effective measures that can prevent or slow the progress of AS. Goals of treatment are: to relieve pain through the use of NSAIDs and heat, for example; to maintain the best possible posture, if necessary with the help of a back brace or splints, so as to prevent breathing problems, and taking short periods of rest to counteract fatigue and maximise energy reserves.

Appropriate exercise to help maintain strength and mobility is advised.

Surgery is rarely necessary to correct deformity of the lumbar spine.

Facet joint injury

Facet joints (page 12) are paired synovial joints at the back of the vertebrae. The capsules of the joints are richly supplied with nerve endings and pain fibres that are sensitive to strain, pressure and stretching.

Like other joints, facet joints are prone to injury and are a not uncommon source of low back pain

Symptoms

Pain both local and referred, muscle spasm and tenderness, and reduced spinal flexibility are the chief symptoms of facet joint injury. Pain is usually worse on extension of the spine and less with flexion.

Causes

Any force that stretches the capsule surrounding a facet joint, and also the ligaments, beyond their tolerance can induce an inflammatory response, resulting in joint pain and swelling.

Prevention
- Regular practise of stretching and strengthening exercises
- Frequent breaks from repetitive work to do tension-relieving exercises
- Posture training, such as that provided by the Alexander Technique

Treatments

Anti-inflammatory medications such as NSAIDs and aspirin may be taken to relieve pain and inflammation.

In selected cases, injection of a steroid such as cortisone directly into the affected joint (page 37) may be an option. This treatment may be useful, for example, when the symptoms are produced by an inflammatory arthritis. One or two repeat injections may be necessary. The efficacy of this therapy for facet joint pain is controversial, however.

Spondylolisthesis

From the Greek *spondylos*, vertebra, and *olisthanein*, to slip, spondylolisthesis refers to a condition in which one vertebra slips over another. This most commonly occurs between the fifth lumbar and the first sacral vertebrae.

Symptoms

Although the spinal instability caused by spondylolisthesis in adults may produce no symptoms, it can sometimes result in back pain. When the condition causes a stenosis, or narrowing in the spinal canal, it can generate symptoms of nerve compression (see spinal stenosis, page 116).

Causes

Arthritic changes in the lumbar spine, most common in older women, are one cause of spondylolisthesis. This can result in a narrowing of the spinal canal.

This condition is also sometimes seen in adolescents and may cause back pain, tight hamstring muscles and nerve irritation.

Prevention

Preventive measures include:
- Regular practise of exercises to strengthen the back and prevent tightness of the hamstring muscles
- Careful attention to posture, body mechanics and correct technique in sports
- Avoiding being overweight

Treatments

Spondylolisthesis due to degenerative changes is treated along lines similar to those for spinal stenosis and for osteoarthritis (page 120). Other treatments include:
- Appropriate stretching and strengthening exercises
- Postural education
- Avoiding becoming overweight
- Not smoking
- Nutritional therapies
- Anti-inflammatory medicines, if necessary
- Injection therapy (page 37), sometimes

Surgical treatments, when considered necessary, consist of decompression and spinal fusion (page 39).

Discs

Between the weight-bearing parts of vertebrae, from the second cervical to the sacrum, are intervertebral discs. They consist of an outer fibrous ring (annulus fibrosus, or AF) and a soft inner substance (nucleus pulposus, or NP). See page 12 for more details. Although the discs can withstand tremendous compression, they do not tolerate rotational stress very well. To compensate, the facet joints help to resist excessive twisting forces.

Degenerative Disc Disease (DDD)

Disc degeneration is a rapid progression of changes in the discs that result in a loss of their integrity and in their ability to distribute load.

Degenerative changes in the spinal discs should not be equated with ageing. Although all discs age, they do not necessarily degenerate.

Symptoms

Degeneration of intervertebral discs does not always produce symptoms. When it does, it can cause a great deal of pain, which worsens with flexion.

Causes

Included in the possible causes of DDD are:
- Excessive force applied to vertebrae through heavy lifting, for example
- Cracks and tears in the AF and leaking from the NP (see above)
- Injury to the discs by excessive pressure, which may be aggravated by rotational forces. The combination can result in an AF tear, which in turn can induce disc herniation

Prevention

Preventive measures include:
- Using correct techniques when exercising and lifting heavy objects
- Using appropriate protective gear when working with vibrating equipment
- Taking periodic relaxation breaks when driving long distances
- Avoiding being overweight

Treatments

As for many other disorders of the spine, therapy for DDD should include:
- Stretching and strengthening exercises
- Training in good posture and body mechanics
- Losing weight if necessary
- Not smoking
- Where appropriate, injection therapy (page 37) and surgery may be considered.

Herniated disc

A weakness in the AF of an intervertebral disc may permit a bulging of the NP; a break or tear allows the NP to protrude or push outward from its normal position. These occurrences, which have given rise to the misnomer 'slipped disc', refer to a herniated disc.

Disc herniation is common among males between the ages of 30 and 50 years and can appear within 36 hours of the precipitating cause.

Symptoms

Among the symptoms occurring with disc herniation are:
- Pain in the back, worsened by flexion and eased by extension
- Pain, numbness and weakness in the legs
- Muscle spasm
- Symptoms suggestive of Cauda Equina Syndrome (page 117)

An entrapped cervical disc undergoes a process similar to that of a herniated disc in the lumbar spine. Symptoms may include neck pain and spasm, changes in sensation in the hand, and a weakened hand grip.

Causes

Changes occurring with the passage of time in both the AF and NP components of spinal discs can contribute to disc herniation.

A fall or other accident, an injury from twisting or lifting, or even an episode of coughing or sneezing can precipitate disc herniation.

Prevention

Sensible preventive measures for minimising the risks of a herniated disc include:

- Regularly engaging in exercises that strengthen the torso, keep the spine flexible and improve balance and coordination
- Taking periodic short breaks from repetitive work to prevent tension build up and unnecessary strain
- Maintaining proper posture at work and elsewhere, to reduce stress on the spine and its components
- Avoiding being overweight
- Wearing proper-fitting low-heeled shoes, to minimise strain on spinal structures

Treatments

Included in the treatments for acute disc herniation, where no red flag symptoms (page 16) appear, are the following:

- Restricted activity but no bed rest, except in severe cases, and then not beyond 48 hours
- Applications of heat to the affected area, to ease muscle spasm and pain

- Medications such as analgesics and anti-inflammatory agents, and cautious use of narcotics
- Gentle exercise (excluding flexion exercises) in consultation with a physiotherapist or other qualified health professional, balanced with periods of relaxation
- Good habits of posture and body mechanics

Steroid injection, discectomy and chemonucleolysis (see pages 37–39) are three minimally invasive options to consider in selected cases.

For a mild to moderate cervical disc problem, a soft cervical collar may be prescribed to limit neck mobility.

CAUTION

During the acute phase of disc herniation, chiropractic and massage are not recommended.

Alternative treatments:

- Acupuncture may be considered for pain relief
- Strategies to help stop smoking would be prudent since smoking is believed to be injurious to the health of the discs
- Yoga and T'ai Chi, which are excellent in helping to attain and maintain flexibility, balance and coordination, are two exercise approaches to consider
- For posture education, the Alexander Technique is superb

Abnormal spinal curves

When viewed from the side, the normal spinal column shows four curves (page 10). These curves contribute to the strength of the spine, absorb shock, help us to maintain balance and give a measure of protection from fracture.

Lordosis

In a normal spine, the lumbar curve bulges forwards. When it is exaggerated, it is known as lordosis.

Symptoms

Any departure from the normal condition of one of the body's structures could affect adjacent tissues. Lordosis subjects other spinal components to muscular strain and may therefore lead to fatigue and pain. If spinal discs become involved, additional symptoms may appear (see page 125).

Causes

Poor postural habits over time can lead to lordosis. The habitual wearing of high-heeled shoes may also be a contributing factor since it alters the body's centre of gravity. Lordosis is also often seen in pregnancy, for the same reason (page 135).

Obesity or a large abdominal tumour can also produce this abnormal spinal curvature.

Prevention

Two keys to preventing lordosis are:
- Good habits of posture and body mechanics
- Maintaining the strength of the back and abdomen through regular exercise
- Wearing sensible shoes is an additional prudent preventive measure to take (see also Orthotics, page 29).

Treatments

Prevention is the best treatment for lordosis. In some cases, however, the temporary use of a brace may be required, and in a few selected cases the extreme measure of spinal fusion surgery may be considered.

Kyphosis

Kyphosis, also referred to as humpback or dowager's hump, is the result of excessive curvature of the thoracic spine.

Symptoms

Like other posture defects, kyphosis can cause fatigue and back pain. A severe curvature that affects the functions of the heart, lungs, stomach and intestines can produce symptoms including an irregular heartbeat, difficulty in breathing and problems with digestion and elimination.

Causes

Kyphosis is common in metabolic disorders such as osteoporosis (page 119) and osteomalacia (softening of bones). It is also sometimes associated with muscular dystrophy, a condition in which muscles weaken and waste away.

Prevention

To help prevent posture defects from developing:
- Exercise regularly to keep limbs and torso strong and flexible
- Posture training and practising good habits of posture and body mechanics are crucial
- Maintaining the weight that is ideal for you is a prudent measure to take

Treatments

- An exercise regime to strengthen muscles and ligaments
- Braces may be used to help improve the deformity
- Analgesics or anti-inflammatory medication can be used to relieve pain and symptoms of inflammation
- If the kyphosis is caused by osteoporosis, appropriate therapeutic measures should be taken (page 119)

- If response to these therapies is unsatisfactory, kyphoplasty (page 39) or other surgery may be required

Alternative treatments:
- Physical therapies including applications of heat and cold, ultrasound, electrical nerve stimulation and massage
- Alexander Technique or other methods of posture training
- Yoga or T'ai Chi for exercises in stretching, strengthening, balance, coordination and relaxation
- Chiropractic for corrective manipulation and strengthening exercise

Scoliosis

Scoliosis is lateral (side-to-side) curvature of the spine in any area. The most common form appears in adolescents and preadolescents.

Symptoms
Apart from possible backache and fatigue resulting from the muscular imbalance caused by scoliosis, breathing difficulties and heart irregularities can appear if the ribcage is seriously deformed.

Causes
Scoliosis can be present at birth (congenital) or due to neuromuscular (nerve-muscle) conditions or spinal trauma.

Treatments
Regular monitoring, preferably by an orthopaedic specialist, is useful in detecting any worsening of the condition.
Non-surgical treatments include:
- Exercise, including swimming and horseback riding to strengthen torso muscles and promote good posture.
- The use of braces for several hours a day may be advised, according to individual requirements
- A physiotherapist can help you organise having the heel of one shoe built up to equalise the length of the legs
- Where necessary, appropriate treatment for the condition producing the spinal defect is given

The decision to proceed with surgery is based not only on the ineffectiveness of conservative treatments, but also on whether the patient is willing to undergo a major operation.

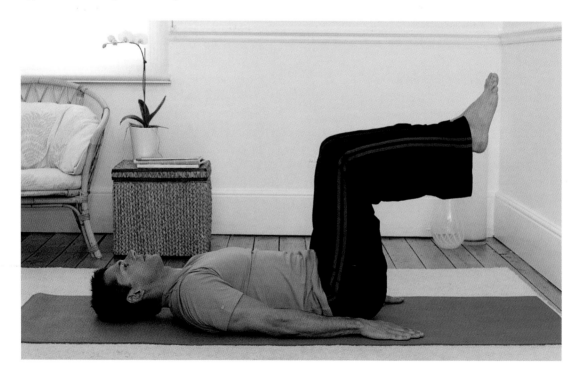

Ligaments and tendons

Ligaments are bands of fibrous tissue that hold bones together. Tendons are fibrous bands that attach muscles to bones. Both can be injured by overstretching, overuse, trauma and poor posture and body mechanics.

Sprains

A sprain is a traumatic injury to the ligaments, tendons or muscles around a joint. In the spine it often affects the ligaments that bind together the facet joints. This occurs most often in the lumbar region, but the sacroiliac joints are sometimes involved.

Symptoms

A sprain usually produces pain, swelling and discolouration of the skin over the affected joint. The pain sometimes radiates to the buttocks and legs. The duration and severity of these symptoms vary with the extent of damage to the supporting tissues.

Causes

Torn or injured ligaments are usually the result of a fall or an activity that produces a wrenching action. They can also be due to overuse, as sometimes occurs in gymnastics or ballet, and from the long-term impact of poor posture and body mechanics.

During pregnancy, when ligaments become lax, some women may be vulnerable to sacroiliac sprain (see page 129).

Prevention

Measures to aid the prevention of sprains include:
- Regular exercise to keep the body strong and flexible
- Frequent breaks from repetitive work to do tension-relieving exercises and so avert cumulative strain
- Good habits of posture and body mechanics
- Warming up adequately before engaging in sports and other vigorous activities (pages 62–73)

Treatments

These include:
- A support device such as a brace, if necessary
- Applications of ice or alternating this with heat
- Ultrasound treatment to help speed up recovery
- Short rest periods, but no prolonged bed rest (which tends to weaken muscles, discs and cartilage, worsen existing back problems and accelerate bone loss)

Muscles

Muscles supporting the spine (page 13) can be vulnerable to a number of injuries including tears, strain and cumulative stress, and also to the development of hard knots called 'trigger points'.

Back strain

Although strain can occur at any level of the spinal column, its most frequent site is the lumbar area. Sometimes the condition is referred to as 'myofascial strain' (myo = muscle; fascia = surrounding tissue).

Symptoms

Pain is one of the first symptoms of back strain and can range in intensity from mild to severe. The pain, which may radiate to the buttocks, usually appears within 36 hours of the precipitating cause, often an injury caused by a fall, a twisting action, or by the lifting of a heavy object. It is aggravated by movement and relieved by rest, and can be worse on flexion of the spine. Muscle spasm may also be present, and there may be localised swelling and tenderness.

Causes

Back strain is usually the result of a minor injury incurred by a fall, a twisting motion, or by incorrectly lifting an object.

Prevention

Keys to helping prevent back strain include:
- Regular practise of stretching and strengthening exercises
- Good habits of posture and body mechanics
- Frequent breaks from repetitive work to practise stress-relieving exercises
- Controlling body weight through sensible nutrition and exercise

Acute-stage treatments (first 48 hours)

In the acute stage, back strain in the lumbar area is best treated with:
- Ice and restricted activity (limited bed rest; gentle stretching exercises and walking)
- Attention to good posture

- Analgesics or anti-inflammatory medicines, if appropriate

Not recommended at this stage are:
- Prolonged bed rest (page 129)
- Application of heat
- Massage
- Braces and other supports

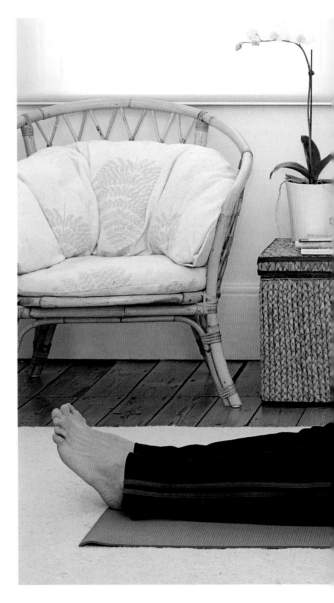

Alternative treatments:
These include: TENS and acupuncture to help speed up rehabilitation, and chiropractic in the absence of radiating pain (as in sciatica with numbness and weakness).

Treatments after 48 hours
Provided that red flag symptoms (page 16) are absent:
- Ultrasound or local applications of heat to reduce spasm, improve function and promote healing
- Ice, following stretching or other suitable exercise

- Prudent use of analgesics or anti-inflammatory medications, with decreasing frequency

Alternative treatments:
- Acupuncture
- Hands-on therapies (pages 30–31) including Shiatsu or other form of massage
- Yoga or T'ai Chi to promote strength, flexibility, balance and coordination

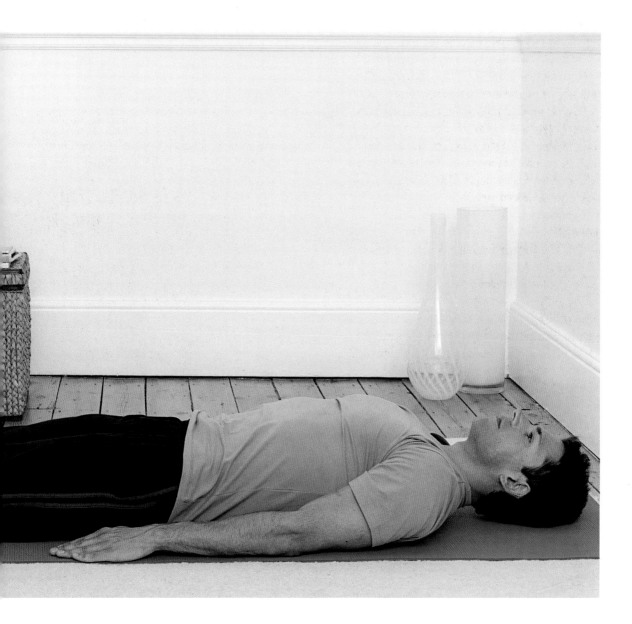

Multiple structures

As mentioned at the start of this chapter, whenever a health disorder occurs, it seldom affects only one part of the body. The neck, or cervical spine, is an example: injury can affect any or all of its bones, joints, nerves, discs, ligaments or muscles. Making the neck even more vulnerable is the fact that it is usually very flexible and capable of a wide range of motion.

Whiplash

Whiplash is a word used to describe certain neck movements under specific conditions. It is a mechanism rather than an injury or illness. It may or may not cause injury.

Symptoms

These vary according to the degree of injury involved. A whiplash movement may produce no symptoms or outward signs of mishap, or it may result in any of the following: neck stiffness and a decrease in the neck's range of motion; tenderness and pain; evidence of neurological injury such as altered sensation and muscle weakness along with pain, or fracture or dislocation of cervical vertebrae, revealed by X-ray. There could also be feelings of dizziness, ringing in the ears and pain in the jaw or arms.

In addition, pain in the cervical spine can spread to the head and produce a headache. This is because the skull is covered by a sheet of muscle that extends from behind it, near the upper neck, to the eyebrows (occipito-frontalis). Tension in the neck can be transmitted to this muscle, which then tightens – much like a drawstring – and can generate a headache.

Causes

Whiplash injury is most often caused by a rear-end car crash that causes the neck of the driver or passenger to be jerked too far backwards (hyperextend) and then too far forwards (hyperflex) and sometimes forwards again. If the vehicle crashes into a stationary object or is involved in a head-on collision, the sequence can be reversed.

Prevention

Although accidents cannot always be prevented, certain measures can be taken to minimise their impact. These include:
- Keeping fit through regular conditioning exercises to keep the body strong, flexible and well toned
- Good habits of posture and body mechanics
- Avoiding being overweight, in order not to stress various body parts unnecessarily

Airbags and properly designed headrests also offer some protection.

Emergency alert

Injury resulting from a whiplash movement could cause fracture and/or dislocation of a vertebra with resulting compression of the spinal cord. This is a medical emergency for which professional help should be summoned immediately: refer to page 16 for appropriate steps to take.

Treatments

Choices of treatment for whiplash injury depend on the individual case. Generally they include:
- Short rest periods while lying on a firm supportive surface
- Gentle neck-stretching exercises for the neck and shoulders as tolerated (check with your doctor or physiotherapist)
- Application of ice alternated with heat, in a 20-minutes on and 20-minutes off cycle
- Pain-relieving or anti-inflammatory medicines as required
- Treatments given by a physiotherapist including: whirlpool baths, hot and cold packs, electrical

nerve stimulation, diathermy, ultrasound or gentle massage
- Taking short, frequent breaks from prolonged sitting (at a desk or computer, for example) to prevent cumulative tension and fatigue
- Surgery may be necessary in some cases of vertebral fracture or dislocation

Alternative treatments:
- Alexander Technique or other posture training method
- Chiropractic or osteopathy in selected cases only (not where osteoporosis is present)
- Relaxation techniques (inherent in methods such as Autogenic Training, biofeedback and yoga)

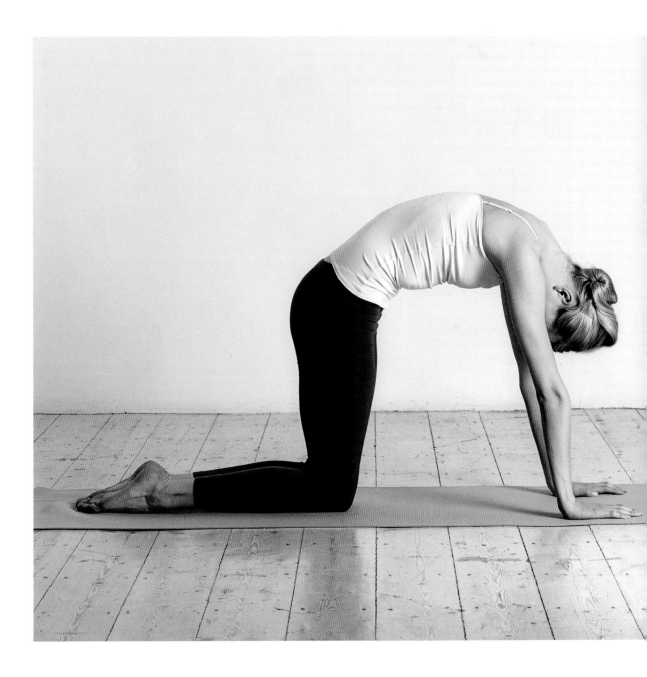

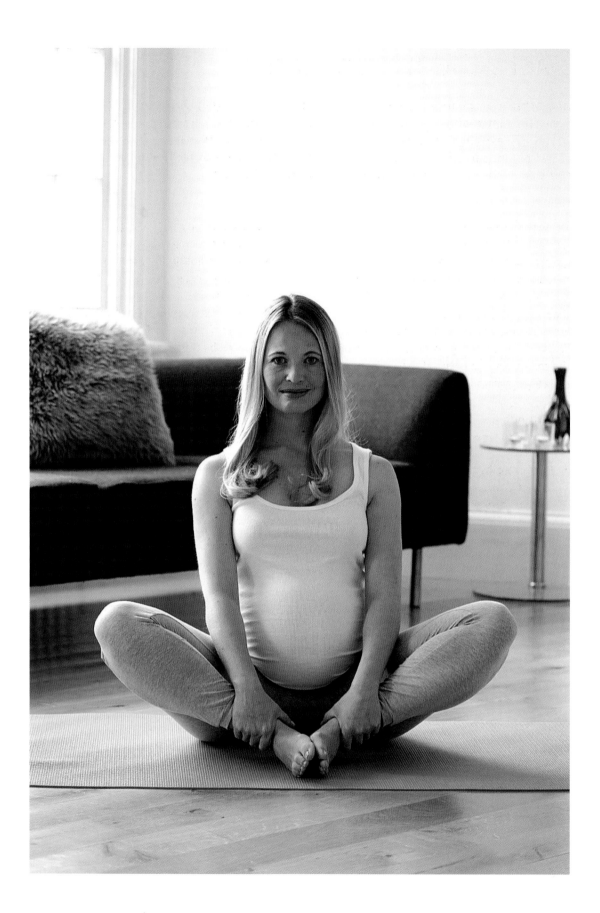

Backache in pregnancy

Backache in pregnancy is a common occurrence and is largely due to a change in the woman's centre of gravity and to the effects of a hormone called relaxin. Relaxin literally relaxes ligaments that support joints, particularly where the spine meets the sacral bones (sacroiliac joints). This is one of nature's ways of facilitating an increase in the size of the passageway to accommodate the child's birth.

As pregnancy progresses and the weight that the woman carries in front increases, her centre of gravity is altered. To compensate, the back muscles have to work harder to help her maintain balance. The pelvis tilts farther forwards and this increases the curve of the lumbar spine (lordosis). Facet joints become strained and in turn further stress ligaments, thus creating a vicious circle. Among the consequences are pain of varying intensity and sometimes symptoms of sciatica (page 116).

Prevention

There are many ways in which to avoid backache in pregnancy:

- Possibly the best preventive measure to take is to keep physically fit. Regularly engaging in appropriate exercise, approved by a doctor, physiotherapist or other health professional, is the key. Exercise helps keep the joints freely moving and strengthens spinal and associated structures to enable you to bear the increased weight of pregnancy with a minimum of discomfort
- Practising good habits of posture and body mechanics (pages 42–55) is also crucial to a largely problem-free pregnancy
- So is taking short periodic breaks from work to do tension-relieving stretches
- Daily relaxation is imperative to guard against accumulated fatigue, which can aggravate pain and other stressors
- Do wear well-fitting low-heeled shoes, which do not further alter your centre of gravity
- Wear a well-fitting bra that supports your enlarging breasts, helps you to maintain good posture and minimises the chances of backache

Non-spinal causes of back pain

Apart from the conditions discussed in the previous pages, many others not originating from the spine itself can give rise to back pain and associated symptoms (see page 16).

You can learn more about these disorders from some of the works mentioned in the bibliography, and from several other sources, including your health-care provider.

It is imperative that you consult a qualified health professional about any pain or troublesome symptoms you experience. He or she will investigate to determine their source and prescribe or recommend appropriate treatment.

Sympathetic nervous system Subdivision of the autonomic nervous system, concerned with processes involving energy expenditure.

Syndrome Group of symptoms typical of a particular disease.

Synovial Pertaining to the lubricating fluid of joints.

Tendon Band of fibrous tissue forming the end of a muscle and attaching it to a bone.

TENS see Transcutaneous Electrical Nerve Stimulation.

Thoracic Pertaining to the chest.

Torsion Twisting.

Transcutaneous Electrical Nerve Stimulation (TENS) The therapeutic application of electrical stimulation to nerves and muscles. Sometimes referred to simply as electrical nerve stimulation.

Tuberculosis (TB) A chronic infection caused by the tubercle bacillus (Koch's bacillus). Diagnosis is based on the results of various tests including sputum culture, X-rays and a tuberculin skin test.

Vertebrae Bones forming the spinal column. Singular: vertebra.

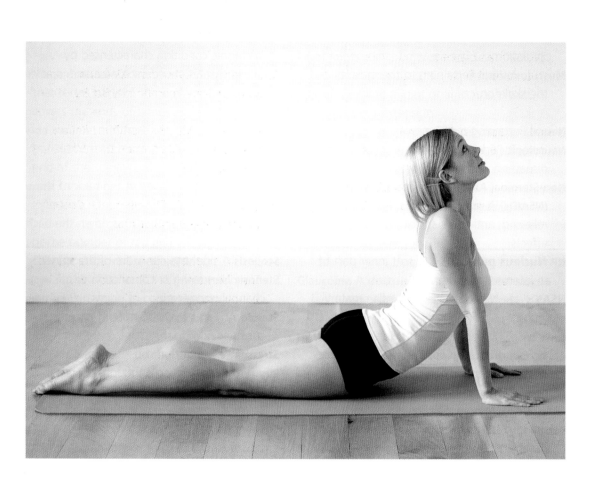

Bibliography

Anderson, Kenneth N., Anderson, Lois E., and Glanze, Walter D. *Mosby's Medical Nursing & Allied Health Dictionary* (5th ed.). St. Louis: Mosby, 1998.

Benson, Herbert, MD. *The Mind/Body Effect*. New York: Simon and Schuster, 1979.

Berkow, Robert, MD, Beers, Mark H., MD, and Fletcher, Andrew J., MD, B.Chir. (Eds). *The Merck Manual of Medical Information* (Home Ed.). New York: Pocket Books, 1997.

Black, Joyce M., PhD, RN, CPSN, CCCN, CWCN, Hawks, Jane Hokanson, DNSc, MSN, RN, C, and Keene, Annabelle M., MSN, RN, C. *Medical-Surgical Nursing. Clinical Management for Positive Outcomes* (6th ed.). Philadelphia: W.B. Saunders, 2001.

Burn, Loic. *Back and Neck Pain. The Facts*. Oxford: Oxford University Press, 2000.

Cailliet, Rene, MD. *Pain: Mechanisms and Management*. Philadelphia: F.A. Davis, 1993.

Cailliet, Rene, MD. *Understand Your Backache*. Philadelphia: F.A. Davis, 19984.

Carrière, Beate. *The Swiss Ball*. Berlin: Springer-Verlag, 1998.

Credit, Larry, P., OMD, Hartunian, Sharon G., LICSW, and Norwak, Margaret J. *Your Guide to Complementary Medicine*. Garden City, New York: Avery Publishing Group, 1998.

Dillard, James, MD, DC, C.Ac., and Ziporyn, Terra, PhD. *Alternative Medicine for Dummies*. Foster City, California: IDG. Books Worldwide, 1998.

Fehrsen-Du Toit, Renita. *The Good Back Book*. Buffalo, New York: Firefly Books, 2003.

Filler, Aaron G., MD, PhD, FRCS (SN). *Do You Really Need Back Surgery?* New York: Oxford University Press, 2004.

Flett, Maureen. *Swiss Ball*. London: PRC Publishing, 2003

Goldenberg, Lorne, and Twist, Peter. *Strength Ball Training*. Champaign, Illinois: Human Kinetics, 2002.

Gray, Henry, FRS. *Anatomy, Descriptive and Surgical*. New York: Bounty Books, 1977.

Hall, Hamilton, MD, FRCSC. *Consultation With the Back Doctor*. Toronto: McClelland & Stewart, 2003.

Hall, Hamilton, MD. *The New Back Doctor*. Toronto: Seal Books, 1995.

Jespersen, Michael, and Potvin, Andre Noel. *The Great Body Ball Handbook*. Blaine, Washington: Productive Fitness Products, 2000.

McCaffery, Margo, RN, MS, FAAN, and Beebe, Alexandra, RN, MS, OCN. *Pain: Clinical Manual for Nursing Practice*. St Louis: The C.V. Mosby Company, 1989.

Melzack, Ronald, and Wall, Patrick D. *The Challenge of Pain.* New York: Basic Books, 1983.

Moffat, Marilyn, PT, PhD, FAPTA, and Vickery, Steve. *The American Physical Therapy Association Book of Body Maintenance and Repair.* New York: Henry Holt, 1999.

Montagu, Ashley. *Touching. The Human Significance of the Skin* (3rd ed.). New York: Harper & Row, 1986.

Noble, Elizabeth, RPT. *Essential Exercises for the Childbearing Year.* Boston: Houghton Mifflin, 1976.

Peddie, Sandra, with Rosenberg, Craig H., MD. *The Repetitive Strain Injury Sourcebook.* Los Angeles: Lowell House, 1997.

Pelletier, Dr. Kenneth R. *The Best Alternative Medicine.* New York: Simon & Schuster, 2000.

Peters, Dr David, and Woodham, Anne. *Natural Health Complete Guide to Integrative Medicine.* London: Dorling Kindersley, 2000.

Reader's Digest Project Staff. *Complete Guide to Pain Relief.* Pleasantville, New York: The Reader's Digest Association, 2000.

Reed, Dr Stephen, MD, FRCSC, and Kendall-Reed, Penny, MSc, ND, with Ford, Dr Michael, MD, FFRCSC, and Gregory, Dr. Charles, MD, ChB, FRCP (C). *The Complete Doctor's Healthy Back Bible.* Toronto: Robert Rose, 2004.

Silverman, Gerald M., DC. *Your Miraculous Back.* Oakland, California: New Harbinger Publications, 2006.

Stuart, Gail W., PhD, RN, CS, FAAN, and Laraia, Michele T., PhD, RN, CS. *Stuart & Sundeen's Principles and Practice of Psychiatric Nursing* (6th ed.). St. Louis: Mosby-Year Book, Inc., 1998.

Sutcliffe, Dr Jenny, MCSP. *The Body Maintenance Manual.* London: The Reader's Digest Association, 1999.

Sutcliffe, Dr. Jenny. *Solving Back Problems.* London: Marshall Editions, 1998.

Thomas, Clayton L., MD, MPH. *Taber's Cyclopedic Medical Dictionary* (15th ed.). Philadelphia: F.A. Davis, 1986.

Tortora, Gerard J., and Grabowski, Sandra Reynolds. *Principles of Anatomy and Physiology* (9th ed.). New York: John Wiley & Sons, 2000.

Weller, Stella. *Healing Yoga.* London: Collins & Brown, 2007.

Winter, Robert B., MD, Back, Marilyn L., PhD, and The Twin Cities Spine Center. *Living Well With Back Pain.* New York: HarperCollins, 2006.

Woodham, Anne, and Peters, Dr David. *Encyclopedia of Healing Therapies.* London: Dorling Kindersley, 1997.

Index

Acknowledgements & Picture Credits

Many thanks to everyone who has contributed to this book. I am particularly grateful to Victoria Alers-Hankey for initiating the project, Miriam Hyslop, Commissioning Editor, with whom I have had an excellent working relationship, and Barbara Dixon, who edited the book.

Special thanks go to Walter for his invaluable assistance at every stage of the work and to David for so unselfishly sharing his time and computer expertise. Thanks also to Karl and Lora for their ongoing interest and support.

Photographs:
page 4 far right Guy Hearn; 10 iStock; 39 Getty; 57 Guy Hearn
All other photography by Dan Duchars